Acknowledgments

Work Group Members

Joy F. Reed, EdD, RN, Chairperson
Betty Bekemeier, MSN, MPH, RN
Kaye Bender, RN, PhD, FAAN
M. Beth Benedict, Dr.P.H., J.D., RN
Ellen L. Bridge, BS, MT, RN
Stephanie Chalupka, EdD, APRN, BC, FAAOHN
Mary Pat Couig, MPH, RN, FAAN
Philip A. Greiner, DNSc, RN
Glenda Kelly, MSN, RN
Joan Kub, PhD, APRN, BC
Pamela A. Kulbok, DNSc, APRN, BC
Deborah S. Martz, BSN, RN

ANA Staff

Carol J. Bickford, PhD, RN, BC—Content editor
Yvonne Daley Humes, MSA—Project coordinator
Matthew Seiler, RN, Esq.—Legal counsel

Winifred Carson-Smith, JD—Legal consultant

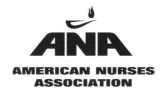

AMERICAN NURSES ASSOCIATION

PUBLIC HEALTH NURSING:
SCOPE AND STANDARDS
OF PRACTICE

nurses
books
.org

The Publishing Program of ANA

AMERICAN NURSES ASSOCIATION
SILVER SPRING, MARYLAND
2007

Library of Congress Cataloging-in-Publication data

Public health nursing : scope and standards of practice /American Nurses Association.
    p. ; cm.
  Includes bibliographical references and index.
  ISBN-13: 978-1-55810-246-0 (pbk.)
  ISBN-10: 1-55810-246-9 (pbk.)
    1. Public health nursing.   2. Community health nursing.   3. Public health
nursing—Practice.   4. Public health nursing—Study and teaching.   I. American
Nurses Association.
  [DNLM: 1. Public Health Nursing—standards—Guideline.   2. Community Health
Nursing—Guideline.   3. Nurse's Role—Guideline. WY 108 P9768 2007]

RT97.P8376 2007
  610.73'4—dc22   2006101337

The American Nurses Association (ANA) is a national professional association. This ANA publication— *Public Health Nursing: Scope and Standards of Practice*—reflects the thinking of the nursing profession on various issues and should be reviewed in conjunction with state board of nursing policies and practices. State law, rules, and regulations govern the practice of nursing, while *Public Health Nursing: Scope and Standards of Practice* guides nurses in the application of their professional skills and responsibilities.

Published by Nursesbooks.org
The Publishing Program of ANA

American Nurses Association
8515 Georgia Avenue, Suite 400
Silver Spring, MD 20910-3492
1-800-274-4ANA
http://www.nursesbooks.org/

ANA is the only full-service professional organization representing the nation's 2.9 million Registered Nurses through its 54 constituent member associations. ANA advances the nursing profession by fostering high standards of nursing practice, promoting the economic and general welfare of nurses in the workplace, projecting a positive and realistic view of nursing, and lobbying the Congress and regulatory agencies on healthcare issues affecting nurses and the public.

Page design: Scott Bell, Arlington, VA ~ *Cover design*: Freedom by Design, Alexandria, VA ~ *Composition*: House of Equations, Inc., Arden, NC ~ *Proofreading*: Lisa Munsat Anthony, Chapel Hill, NC ~ *Editing & Indexing*: Steven A. Jent, Denton, TX ~ *Printing*: McArdle Printing, Upper Marlboro, MD

First printing December 2006.   Second Printing July 2007.

ISBN-13: 978-1-55810-246-0   SAN: 851-3481
5M 07/07R

Contents

PREFACE

Public Health Nursing: Scope and Standards of Practice outlines the expectations of the professional role within which all public health registered nurses should practice. This scope statement and these updated standards of public health nursing practice are meant to guide, define, and direct public health professional nursing practice in all settings.

The American Nurses Association (ANA) has actively engaged in scope of practice and standards development initiatives since the late 1960s. ANA published the first *Standards of Nursing Practice* for the nursing profession in 1973. The standards were generic in nature and focused on the basic nursing process—a critical thinking model applicable to all registered nurses—composed of assessment, diagnosis, outcomes identification, planning, implementation, and evaluation. Over the years, various revisions have ensued, the most recent being *Nursing: Scope and Standards of Practice* (ANA, 2004). Specialty nursing organizations have affirmed this work by using the template language of the standards when developing scope of practice statements and standards of practice for registered nurses engaged in specialty practice.

The Quad Council of Public Health Nursing Organizations, which represents nurses involved in population-focused and community-oriented nursing practice, collaborated with ANA over several years to create *Scope and Standards of Public Health Nursing Practice* (Quad Council & ANA, 1999). This effort was intended to help meet the growing demand for healthcare professionals dedicated to health promotion and protection services for individuals and populations. Since that time, significant national and global events, such as the HIV/AIDs epidemic, natural disasters, and terrorist attacks within the United States, have intensified individual and population concerns.

As part of its regular scope and standards of nursing practice development, review, and maintenance processes, the ANA convened a volunteer work group of public health and community health nursing stakeholders in 2004 to review and revise the 1999 *Scope and Standards of Public Health Nursing Practice* to best reflect contemporary public health nursing practice and set a framework for future practice. ANA specifically charged this work group to review and incorporate relevant content from the 1986 *Standards of Community Health Nursing*. After careful review and consideration, the work group determined that the 2006 *Public Health Nursing: Scope and Standards of Practice* would fully incorporate and replace that 1986 document. The work group also made a conscious decision to use *Advanced Practice Public Health Nurse* to denote the second level of practice (i.e., clinical nurse specialist). This is consistent with and reinforces the ANA position that the clinical nurse specialist is one of the four advanced practice roles in nursing.

The work group:

- analyzed numerous reports and publications of the Institute of Medicine (IOM), the American Public Health Association (APHA), and other organizations as part of an environmental assessment,

- sought comment on a draft model and standards from attendees at a special forum at the 2004 fall APHA meeting,

- notified ANA's constituent member associations, specialty nursing organizations, public health organizations, and other stakeholders that input was requested on the draft document,

- posted the draft document on ANA's www.NursingWorld.org web site for public review and comment by interested nurses and others,

- considered all public suggestions posted during the comment period, and

- finalized the draft document for submission to the ANA review and publication process.

The ANA review included evaluation by the Committee on Nursing Practice Standards and Guidelines of ANA's Congress on Nursing Practice and Economics for compliance with established criteria. The Congress on Nursing Practice and Economics then completed another level of review, culminating in the approval of the specialty scope of practice statement and acknowledgment of the specialty nursing standards of practice.

The goal of public health nursing is to improve the health and well-being of all individuals, families, communities, and populations through the significant and visible contributions of registered nurses utilizing standards-based practice. This goal will be achieved when the contents of this document are consistently applied to practice, education, and research. For example, the scope and standards for public health nursing may be used as the basis for developing public health nursing job descriptions and performance evaluations. In the population-focused nursing education domain, the scope and standards can guide curriculum development. Finally, the rich content of the public health nursing scope and standards of practice can provide direction for expanding the focus of the public health nursing research agenda.

Public Health Nursing: Scope of Practice

Context for Twenty-first Century Public Health Nursing Practice

For over a century, public health nursing has significantly contributed to population-focused health through effective partnerships. Beginning in the early part of the twentieth century, Lillian Wald, Lavinia Dock, and their nursing colleagues at the Henry Street Settlement House in New York's lower East Side applied spirited innovation to organize themselves and others, working in and with communities to heal, partner, mobilize, support, and bring about change in the disadvantaged populations in which they lived and worked. Such partnerships continue today as public health nurses work with communities and populations to identify specific public health assets and needs, addressing those issues at multiple levels, and using the political process to assure the health of communities.

Several reports and events have influenced how public health nurses conceptualize and define the practice of public health nursing for the twenty-first century. The Institute of Medicine's report, *The Future of the Public's Health in the Twenty-first Century* (2003a), builds upon a previous IOM report, *The Future of Public Health* (1988), and contains specific recommendations for strengthening the relationships among the vital sectors charged with protecting the public's health. These sectors include the governmental public health infrastructure, communities (including schools, elected officials, and community and faith-based organizations), healthcare delivery systems, employers and businesses, the media, academia, and the research community.

An ecological approach, proposed by the IOM's 2003 report, is the basis for understanding health in populations. This approach recognizes multiple determinants of health that are critical not only for understanding the concept of health, but also for assuring conditions in which populations may achieve good health. This ecological approach is also based on the assumption that health is influenced at several levels within the ecological framework, such as individuals, families, communities, organizations, and social systems. An ecological approach to public health nursing practice is based on population-focused services and programs, advocacy, research, and education. See Appendix A for a comparison of selected well-known public health nursing intervention models and the multiple determinants of population health using this ecological approach.

Nursing comprises the largest single workforce in the health system. Therefore, nurses have significant opportunities to create an environment that ensures good health. This is especially true in public health nursing practice with its focus on health promotion, disease prevention, and improved health status through nursing care and collaboration with communities. These services and programs often alter the interaction of the determinants of health to produce conditions in which people may attain and maintain health. Recommendations from *The Future of the Public's Health in the Twenty-first Century* (IOM, 2003a) provide direction for defining and creating new approaches in public health nursing practice, education, and research that utilize the ecological model to alter the social determinants of health.

A companion IOM study, *Who Will Keep the Public Healthy?* (2003b), also builds on an ecological approach and considers factors likely to influence public health in the twenty-first century, such as globalization, technological and scientific advances, and demographic shifts in the United States. This IOM report explores issues and lists recommendations regarding further development of the public health workforce. A public health professional is defined in this report as a person educated in public health or a related discipline who is engaged in improving health through a focus on populations.

The report delineates eight new content domains for public health professionals: informatics, genomics, communication, cultural competence, community-based participatory research, policy and law, global health, and ethics. These content areas are proposed to assist the present and future public health workforce to meet the emerging needs of new global public health issues and advances in science and policy. Both IOM reports emphasize the vision of the national health objectives for healthy people in healthy communities as described in *Healthy People 2010* (HHS, 2000; http://www.healthypeople.gov/Publications/).

The development of public health competencies by the Council on Linkages Between Academia and Public Health Practice (2001) is another landmark effort with potential influence on the public health nursing specialty. These competencies provide direction for the education, practice, and future research of public health professionals.

The Quad Council of Public Health Nursing Organizations, an alliance of the Association of Community Health Nursing Educators (ACHNE), the American Nurses Association's (ANA) Congress on Nursing Practice and Economics, the American Public Health Association Public Health Nursing Section, and the Association of State and Territorial Directors of Nursing (ASTDN), developed public health nursing specific competencies (Quad Council of Public Health Nursing Organizations, 2004), using the Council on Linkages competencies as a framework (Council on Linkages Between Academia and Practice, 2001). These public health nursing competencies were designed to be used with other documents, such as *The Definition and Role of Public Health Nursing* (APHA PHN Section, 1996) and the 1999 edition of the *Scope and Standards of Public Health Nursing Practice* (Quad Council & ANA, 1999). The public health nursing competencies called attention to the population-focused nature of public health nursing practice and emphasized how public health nursing is unique in its approach to health improvement at the individual, family, community, and population levels.

Another set of documents to be considered in guiding the work of public health nursing for the twenty-first century is the *National Public Health Performance Standards* (CDC, 2001). These standards define optimal performance at the state, local, and federal levels of public health and are designed to guide self-assessment and quality improvement activities for the operation of public health systems well into the future. For the NPHPS assessment, the public health system is defined in its broadest context, similar to the ecological model used in the 2003 IOM report, and considers all partners with a role in improving and protecting the public's health.

Public health nursing practice in the United States is becoming increasingly complex. Societal and political changes have contributed to this complexity. Threats to the health of populations include a re-emergence of communicable diseases, increasing incidence of drug-resistant organisms, overall concern about the structure of the healthcare system, environmental hazards, and the challenges imposed by the presence of modern public health epidemics such as obesity- and tobacco-related deaths.

Global and emerging crises have increased the vulnerability of populations to multiple health threats. These threats have dramatically redirected attention toward public health preparedness with its new priorities and activities, such as syndromic surveillance, mass casualty planning, and the handling of biological and chemical agents as evidentiary material as well as for removal of a public health hazard. Postal workers, law enforcement personnel, and communications experts are among the new groups that have emerged as partners with public health nurses (IOM, 1995).

Public health nurses exhibit leadership in many of these emerging priority public health initiatives. These roles provide opportunities for public health nurses to determine the evidence by which new public health system changes are implemented and evaluated, and then to develop operational systems that can be effectively deployed for any emerging public health threat. Similarly, public health nurses are also increasingly identified as leaders in public health system reform.

During the twenty-first century there is likely to be an even greater emphasis on population-focused services in public health demanding new knowledge and skills of public health nurses. The practice of public health nurses of this century will be guided not only by sound application of evidence-based intervention models, but also by these sources

- Current scope and standards of practice for public health nursing
- Core functions of public health (IOM, 1988)
- Ten Essential Public Health Services (http://www.cdc.gov/od/ocphp/nphpsp/EssentialPHServices.htm)
- *Definition and Role of Public Health Nursing* (APHA, 1996)
- Quad Council Public Health Nursing Competencies (2004)
- *Healthy People 2010,* (HHS, 2000)
- *National Public Health Performance Standards* (CDC, 2001)
- *Essentials of Baccalaureate Nursing Education for Entry Level Community Health Nursing Practice* (ACHNE, 2000)
- *Essentials of Master's Level Nursing Education for Advanced Community/Public Health Nursing Practice* (ACHNE, 2003)
- An ecological approach model similar to that described in *The Future of the Public's Health in the Twenty-first Century* (IOM, 2003a).

Definition of Public Health Nursing

Public health nursing is the practice of promoting and protecting the health of populations using knowledge from nursing, social, and public health sciences (American Public Health Association, Public Health Nursing Section, 1996). The practice is population-focused with the goals of promoting health and preventing disease and disability for all people through the creation of conditions in which people can be healthy.

Although practicing in a variety of public and private organizations, all public health nurses focus on one or more populations. A population may be defined as those living in a specific geographic area (e.g., a neighborhood, community, city or county) or those in a particular group (e.g., racial, ethnic, age, disease) who experience a disproportionate burden of poor health outcomes.

Population-based public health nursing practice focuses on entire populations that possess similar health concerns or characteristics. This includes everyone in a population who is actually or potentially affected by a health concern or shares a specific characteristic. Population-based public health nursing interventions are not limited to those who seek service, are poor, or otherwise vulnerable. Public health nursing services and programs may be directed toward entire populations within a community, the systems that affect the health of those populations, or the individuals and families within those populations. The public health nurse partners with communities and populations to reduce health risks and to promote, maintain, and restore health, advocating for system-level changes to improve health.

Public health nurses must understand and apply concepts from various disciplines, including community organization and development, coordination of care, health education and maintenance, and environmental health, in addition to nursing and public health sciences. Public health nurses practice in partnership with the population and numerous other groups, including:

- members of the public health team such as epidemiologists, social workers, nutritionists, environmental health workers, and health educators;
- local, state, and federal public health organizations;
- healthcare providers;

- community organizations and coalitions;
- community service agencies such as schools, law enforcement, and emergency response;
- faith-based organizations;
- businesses and industries; and
- academic and research institutions.

Public health nurses work to improve health at the individual, family, community, and population levels through the core functions of assessment, assurance, and policy development (IOM, 1988). The core functions are applied in a systematic and comprehensive manner.

Assessment includes a review of the concerns, strengths and expectations of the population and is guided by epidemiological methods and the nursing process.

Assurance is accomplished through regulation, advocating for other healthcare professionals to provide needed services, coordinating community services, or, at times, direct provision of services. Assurance strategies take into account the availability, acceptability, accessibility, and quality and effectiveness of services. Public health nurses focus on assurance activities and initiatives that provide appropriate service delivery to achieve targeted outcomes and that monitor health service access, utilization, and appropriateness for the community, including underserved and target populations. In addition, assurance functions include participation in developing systems and programs to promote positive health outcomes for the community, working to implement continuous quality improvement for healthcare systems in the community, and providing expert public health nurse consultation to groups and organizations in the community.

The necessary policies are developed according to the results of the assessment, the priorities set by the population, and consideration of subpopulations and communities at greatest risk, as well as the evidence on effectiveness of various activities or strategies.

Public health nurses are proactive with respect to social and healthcare trends, changing concerns, and policy and legislative activities. They function as advocates for the populations they serve. Such advocacy for public health and social policies promotes a healthy environment, creates conditions that improve and enhance the health of populations, and is a key part of public health nursing roles.

Public health nurses engage in research that enhances public health nursing practice and documents the outcomes of specific activities and strategies. They have an obligation to actively enhance the science and evidence base for professional practice. A clear and well-documented evidence base for public health nursing practice permits the use of the most efficient, effective, and cost-beneficial strategies in promoting the public's health.

When public health nurses partner with individuals, the focus becomes the promotion of knowledge, attitudes, beliefs, practices, and behaviors that support and enhance health, with the ultimate goal of improving the overall health of the population. Similarly, activities with families and communities aim at promoting family and community norms, attitudes, awareness, and behaviors that improve the family's or community's overall health. Activities with populations address organizations, policies, and laws, and include key stakeholders that affect the environment in which people reside and create conditions which allow or promote health for all.

Distinguishing Public Health Nursing from Other Nursing Specialties

Public health nurses enter the specialty from diverse educational and practice backgrounds. While public health nursing practice is traditionally associated with nurses employed by governmental agencies, such as state, local, and tribal health departments, the work also occurs in settings such as community- or faith-based organizations, health maintenance organizations, and community health centers. For purposes of this document, the definition of a public health professional cited in *Who Will Keep the Public Healthy?* describes the work of public health nurses, regardless of their employment setting: "A public health professional is a person educated in public health or a related discipline who is employed to improve health through a population focus" (IOM, 2003b).

Grounded in both the nursing and the public health sciences, public health nursing is distinguished from other nursing specialties by its adherence to *all* of the following eight principles:

- *The client or* unit of care *is the population.* While a public health nurse may engage in activities with individuals, families, or groups, the dominant responsibility is to the population as a whole.

- *The primary obligation is to achieve the greatest good for the greatest number of people or the population as a whole.* Public health nurses recognize that it may not be possible to meet individual needs if those needs conflict with priority health goals that benefit the whole population.

- *The processes used by public health nurses include working with the client as an equal partner.* The public health nurse's actions must reflect awareness of the need for comprehensive health planning in partnership with communities and populations and include the perspectives, priorities, and values of the population in interpreting the data, making policy and program decisions, and selecting appropriate strategies for action.

- *Primary prevention is the priority in selecting appropriate activities.* Primary prevention includes health promotion and health protection strategies.

- *Public health nursing focuses on strategies that create healthy environmental, social, and economic conditions in which populations may thrive.* Public health nursing interventions include education, community development, social engineering, policy development, and enforcement. Such interventions emerge from work with the population and result in laws and rules, policies, and budget priorities. Advocating for and teaching advocacy skills to others to create healthy conditions is an essential part of public health nursing practice.

- *A public health nurse is obligated to actively identify and reach out to all who might benefit from a specific activity or service.* Because risk factors are not randomly distributed, specific subpopulations may be more vulnerable to disease or disability or may have more difficulty in accessing or using services, thus requiring special outreach. Public health nurses focus on the whole population and not just those who present for services.

- *Optimal use of available resources to assure the best overall improvement in the health of the population is a key element of the practice.* Public health nurses must be involved in organizing and coordinating the actions of others in response to health issues. In addition, they must use and provide information to other decision-makers regarding the scientific evidence related to outcomes of specific actions, programs, or policies, as well as the cost-effectiveness of potential strategies. Public health nurses must also strive to create the evidence where it is lacking.

- *Collaboration with a variety of other professions, populations, organizations, and other stakeholder groups is the most effective way to promote and protect the health of the people.* Creating the conditions in which people can be healthy is an extremely complex, resource-intensive process. Public health nurses join with appropriate experts from a variety of fields and professions, as well as community members, in efforts to improve population health. This includes public health nurses' recognition of the importance of legislative action and involvement in other means by which health and social policies are set at all levels. This collaboration may occur within the healthcare system or the government; it promotes adoption or revision of such policies.

Ethical Responsibilities

Public health nurses are bound by the ethical provisions for all nurses made explicit in *Code of Ethics for Nurses with Interpretive Statements* (ANA, 2001), *Principles of Ethical Practice of Public Health* (Public Health Leadership Society, 2002), and *Environmental Health Principles and Recommendations for Public Health Nursing* (APHA, 2006). In working with populations, public health nurses must acknowledge the right of the population to have access to the necessary information and opportunities for dialogue in order to make informed decisions without coercion.

Advances in scientific, medical, and healthcare technologies create ethical and legal questions that must be addressed while respecting the diverse values, beliefs, and cultures present in the population served. The need to receive or share information concerning an individual's health in order to protect the health of the public creates a unique set of ethical issues for public health nurses. Likewise, the promise of genomics for contributing to the understanding of and ability to prevent morbidity and mortality must be tempered by the possibility of using such information to further disenfranchise and limit access to care for certain populations.

The purpose of public health nursing science is to enhance the health of populations. Public health nurses must recognize and establish their professional practice in accordance with the populations' rights and with a particular concern for social justice. This includes using the Precautionary Principle to guide practice and engage in preventive actions in the face of uncertainty, exploring a wide range of alternatives to potentially harmful actions, and promoting increased public participation in decision-making (Tickner, 2002; Tickner & Raffensberger, 1998). In addition, when making decisions that have an impact on health, public health nurses are obligated to assure that ethical issues are addressed as part of the decision-making process. Public health nurses should also be represented on ethics bodies that make decisions that affect the rights of the population and public health nurses.

Education

The baccalaureate degree in nursing is the educational credential for entry into public health nursing practice. Master's level education is assumed for the nurse specialist level with specific expertise in population-focused care. This educational preparation best prepares public health nurses to function in the specialty role. Associate degree and diploma-prepared registered nurses and licensed practical nurses may appropriately practice in community settings where care is directed toward the health or illness of individuals or families, rather than populations.

In the accompanying standards of practice, the term *advanced practice public health nurse* is used to describe the additional expectations of master's-prepared public health nurses who function as clinical nurse specialists or nurse practitioners in population-focused care (ANA, 2003, 2004a). This advanced practice registered nurse must meet all of the educational and practice criteria required for both generalist and specialist public health nursing practice. Public health nurses who function in nurse administrator roles should additionally use *Scope and Standards for Nurse Administrators* (ANA, 2004b).

Many public health nursing roles require knowledge, skills, and abilities at the doctoral level. Multiple venues for pursuing doctoral level education exist, and program selection may depend on the role the public health nurse holds or wishes to hold (e.g., clinical practice or research, interdisciplinary public health, informatics, epidemiology, ethics).

The individual public health nurse pursuing a doctorate needs to assure that the population focus is a central component of the selected course of study.

All public health nurses are expected to be lifelong learners. This means they actively engage in a process of self-assessment to review their current knowledge, skills, and abilities to identify areas for further development. Such professional development may include enrollment in a formal academic program or participation in continuing education studies. Specialty certification in public health nursing is available from the American Nurses Credentialing Center (ANCC) for the public health/community health clinical nurse specialist.

Summary

Public health nursing has historically responded to the needs of populations through effective partnerships. Promoting and protecting population health in the twenty-first century requires that public health nurses have an understanding of the multiple determinants of health. This ecological approach to health is critical as public health nurses not only respond to the health concerns of individuals and communities, but are proactive in the development and implementation of programs and policies to enhance the health of populations. Public health nursing emphasizes the core functions and essential services of public health. The role of the public health nurse is distinguished from other nursing specialties by its emphasis on population-focused services with goals of promoting health and preventing disease and disability, as well as improving quality of life. Public health nurses work to create environmental conditions to assure health through collaboration with a variety of other professions, organizations, and communities. In the context of an evolving healthcare system for the twenty-first century, public health nurses are valued members of the public health workforce; they have the knowledge and skills to deal with the threats, barriers, and factors that influence the health of populations.

STANDARDS OF PUBLIC HEALTH NURSING PRACTICE

The Standards of Public Health Nursing Practice and the associated measurement criteria are adapted from and reflect the intent of the template language of the Standards of Practice and Standards of Professional Performance presented in *Nursing: Scope and Standards of Practice* (ANA, 2004a).

Standards of Practice

The six Standards of Practice describe a competent level of public health nursing care as demonstrated by the critical thinking model known as the nursing process. The nursing process includes the components of assessment, diagnosis, outcomes identification, planning, implementation, and evaluation. The nursing process encompasses all significant actions taken by registered nurses and forms the foundation of the nurse's decision-making.

Standards of Professional Performance

Taken together the ten Standards of Professional Performance describe competency in the professional role. The standards address a competency level, including activities related to quality of practice, education, professional practice evaluation, collegiality, collaboration, ethics, research, resource utilization, and leadership. The advocacy standard addresses the unique responsibility of all public health nurses to serve as spokespersons for those who cannot address their own healthcare concerns.

Measurement Criteria

Measurement criteria are key indicators of competent practice for each standard. For a standard to be met, all the listed measurement criteria must be met.

Standards should remain stable over time, as they reflect the philosophical values of the profession. Measurement criteria, however, can be revised more frequently to incorporate advancements in scientific knowledge and expectations for nursing practice. Additional measurement criteria that are applicable only to advanced practice registered nurses are included for select standards of practice and professional performance.

Words such as *appropriate* and *possible* are sometimes used because a document like this one cannot account for all situations that the public health nurse may encounter in practice. The registered nurse will need to exercise judgment based on education and experience in determining what is appropriate or possible for a population or situation. Further direction may be available from documents such as guidelines for practice or agency standards, policies, procedures, and protocols.

STANDARDS OF PUBLIC HEALTH NURSING PRACTICE
STANDARDS OF PRACTICE

STANDARD 1. ASSESSMENT
The public health nurse collects comprehensive data pertinent to the health status of populations.

Measurement Criteria:

The public health nurse:

- Collects multi-source data related to the health of the public at large or of a specific population.

- Uses models and principles of epidemiology, demography, and biometry, as well as social, behavioral, and physical sciences to structure data collection.

- Sets assessment priorities based on urgency of need or risk in geographic areas or in populations.

- Conducts an assessment based on criteria that aim to capture the population assets and needs, values and beliefs, resources, and relevant environmental factors.

- Analyzes data using problem-solving techniques and models from nursing, public health, and other disciplines.

- Interprets data to identify trends and deviations from expected health patterns in the population.

- Documents assessment data in terms that are understandable to all involved in the process.

- Applies ethical, legal, and privacy guidelines and policies to the collection, maintenance, use, and dissemination of data and information.

Additional Measurement Criteria for the Advanced Practice Public Health Nurse:

The advanced practice public health nurse:

- Gathers data from multiple, interdisciplinary sources using appropriate methods to augment or verify population-focused data.

Continued ▶

Standards of Public Health Nursing Practice   **15**

- Partners with populations, health professionals, and other stake-holders to attach meaning to collected data.

- Synthesizes complex, multi-source data gathered through the assessment process.

- Consults with the public health nurse, the population, the interdisciplinary team, and other stakeholders in the design, management, and evaluation of the data system that focuses on population assets, needs, and concerns.

STANDARD 2. POPULATION DIAGNOSIS AND PRIORITIES
The public health nurse analyses the assessment data to determine the population diagnoses and priorities.

Measurement Criteria:

The public health nurse:

- Derives the population diagnoses and priorities based on assessment data such as:

  - input from the population,

  - data related to access and use of health services,

  - factors contributing to health promotion and disease prevention,

  - existing or potential harmful exposures, and

  - basic nursing and public health-related sciences.

- Validates the diagnoses or concerns with the population; local, state, and federal public heath agencies and organizations; and available health data and statistics as applicable.

- Documents diagnoses or concerns in a manner that facilitates population involvement in the determination of the plan and its expected outcomes.

Additional Measurement Criteria for the Advanced Practice Public Health Nurse:

The advanced practice public health nurse:

- Organizes complex data and information obtained during sociocultural, demographic, health status and health risk, geographic, environmental, and other nursing and public heath diagnostic processes to identify population health assets, needs, and risks.

- Systematically analyzes relevant population data, scientific principles, and events in the environment in formulating differential diagnoses and in setting priorities.

STANDARD 3. OUTCOMES IDENTIFICATION

The public health nurse identifies expected outcomes for a plan that is based on population diagnoses and priorities.

Measurement Criteria:

The public health nurse:

- Involves the population and other professionals, organizations, and stakeholders in formulating expected outcomes.

- Derives culturally relevant expected outcomes from the diagnoses.

- Considers population values and beliefs, health literacy, risks, benefits, costs, current social policies, current scientific evidence, and expertise when formulating priorities and expected outcomes.

- Incorporates knowledge of environmental factors and events, available resources, time estimates, and ethical, legal, and privacy considerations in defining expected outcomes.

- Develops outcomes that provide continuity in meeting population needs and concerns and enhancing assets.

- Modifies expected outcomes based on changes in population needs or concerns and the availability of resources.

- Documents expected outcomes as measurable objectives using language that is understandable to all involved entities.

- Applies nursing and public health competencies when measuring effective practice in a community or a population.

Additional Measurement Criteria for the Advanced Practice Public Health Nurse:

The advanced practice public health nurse:

- Assures that professional partners are involved in identifying expected outcomes that incorporate scientific evidence and are achievable through implementation of evidence-based practices.

- Assures that measurable outcomes include such factors as cost-effectiveness, satisfaction of stakeholders, the population, and organization, continuity and consistency of services, and resolution of health concerns.

STANDARD 4. PLANNING
The public health nurse develops a plan that reflects best practices by identifying strategies, action plans, and alternatives to attain expected outcomes.

Measurement Criteria:

The public health nurse:

- Assists with the development of population-focused plans for health-related services or programs based on an assessment and prioritization of health assets, needs, risks, and concerns.

- Incorporates evidence-based approaches for promotion, improvement, and restoration of health; prevention of illness, injury, or disease; and emergency preparedness and response that address the identified assets, needs, and concerns.

- Provides for continuity within and across programs and services.

- Establishes plans that reflect cultural competence, educational and learning principles, and priorities that address the population needs.

- Ensures participation of the identified population, health professionals, coalitions, organizations, and other stakeholders in determining roles within the planning processes.

- Applies current standards, statutes, regulations, and policies in the planning process.

- Integrates current and emerging trends and research in nursing and public health-related fields in the planning process.

- Considers the economic impacts of the plan on the population and organizations.

- Documents the plan using language that is culturally sensitive and at an appropriate reading level to be understood by all participants.

- Uses standardized terminology to document the plan.

Additional Measurement Criteria for the Advanced Practice Public Health Nurse:

The advanced practice public health nurse:

- Applies assessment, implementation, and evaluation strategies in the plan to reflect current evidence, including data, research, literature, and expert nursing and public health knowledge.

- Designs appropriate strategies and alternatives with community and professional partners to meet the complex needs of at-risk populations.

- Incorporates population values and beliefs with community and professional partners in the planning process.

- Leads other public health nurses and the multi-sector team in the use of principles of planning for population-focused programs and services.

- Contributes to the development and continuous improvement of organizational systems that support the planning process.

- Participates in the integration of human, fiscal, material, scientific, and population resources to enhance and complete the planning process for programs or services.

- Assures that the current standards, statutes, regulations, and policies are considered in the planning process.

STANDARD 5. IMPLEMENTATION
The public health nurse implements the identified plan by partnering with others.

Measurement Criteria:

The public health nurse:

- Implements the identified plan in a safe and timely manner in collaboration with the multi-sector team.

- Applies evidence-based strategies and activities, including opportunities for coalition building and advocacy, in a plan that is specific to the population assets, needs, and concerns.

- Incorporates systems and population resources in implementing the plan.

- Monitors implementation of the plan, including processes and resource utilization.

- Documents implementation of the plan, including modifications.

Additional Measurement Criteria for the Advanced Practice Public Health Nurse:

The advanced practice public health nurse:

- Interprets surveillance data related to the plan and population health status.

- Incorporates new knowledge and strategies into action plans to enhance implementation.

- Modifies the plan based on new knowledge, appropriate health behavior change theory, population response, or other relevant factors to achieve expected outcomes.

- Advocates for bringing needed resources to the community and for the population to implement the plan.

- Fosters new collaborative relationships with nursing colleagues, other professionals, community or population representatives, and other stakeholders to implement the plan through strategies such as coalition building.

- Promotes organizations, community coalitions, and systems that support the plan.

STANDARD 5A. COORDINATION

The public health nurse coordinates programs, services, and other activities to implement the identified plan.

Measurement Criteria:

The public health nurse:

- Promotes policies, programs, and services for the attainment of expected outcomes.

- Conducts surveillance, case finding, and reporting functions with health professionals and other stakeholders.

- Connects populations with needed services.

- Documents the coordination and required reporting.

Additional Measurement Criteria for the Advanced Practice Public Health Nurse:

The advanced practice public health nurse:

- Provides leadership for delivery of integrated programs, services, and public policy implementation.

- Synthesizes data and information to initiate system, community, and environmental resource allocation that support the delivery of programs and services.

Standard 5b. Health Education And Health Promotion

The public health nurse employs multiple strategies to promote health, prevent disease, and ensure a safe environment for populations.

Measurement Criteria:

The public health nurse:

- Includes appropriate health education in the implementation of programs and services for populations.

- Selects teaching and learning methods appropriate to the health literacy of the population and their identified objectives.

- Presents culturally and age-appropriate health promotion, disease prevention, and environmental safety information and educational materials to the population.

- Collects feedback from participants to determine program and service effectiveness and recommended changes.

Additional Measurement Criteria for the Advanced Practice Public Health Nurse:

The advanced practice public health nurse:

- Provides leadership to nursing and other health professionals in planning evidence-based educational programs and services based on assessments.

- Designs health information and programs based on health behavior, learning theories and principles, and research evidence.

- Modifies existing programs based on feedback from participants, providers, health professionals, and other stakeholders.

- Develops health information resources that are culturally and age-appropriate to the population.

STANDARD 5C. CONSULTATION

The public health nurse provides consultation to various community groups and officials to facilitate the implementation of programs and services.

Measurement Criteria:

The public health nurse:

- Confers with community organizations and groups to facilitate participation in programs and services.

- Provides testimony and professional opinion on programs and service delivery to at-risk populations.

- Communicates effectively using a variety of media with constituent groups during consultation.

- Documents the scope and effectiveness of consultation activities provided to community populations.

Additional Measurement Criteria for the Advanced Practice Public Health Nurse:

The advanced practice public health nurse:

- Synthesizes data from federal, state, local, and other sources with theoretical frameworks and evidence, to provide expert consultation on program and service implementation.

- Provides expert testimony at the federal, state, and local levels on program and service delivery to at-risk populations.

- Communicates information during consultation toward a positive influence on the provision of programs and services to populations.

- Generates proposals and reports in support of needed programs and services.

STANDARD 5D. REGULATORY ACTIVITIES
The public health nurse identifies, interprets, and implements public health laws, regulations, and policies.

Measurement Criteria:

The public health nurse:

- Educates affected populations on relevant laws, regulations, and policies.

- Participates in the application of public health laws, regulations, and policies, including monitoring and inspecting regulated entities.

- Collects specific information about situations that are reported to public health officials.

- Assists in addressing non-compliance with laws, regulations, and policies.

Additional Measurement Criteria for the Advanced Practice Public Health Nurse:

The advanced practice public health nurse:

- Collaborates in the revision or development of public health laws, regulations, and policies.

- Designs, with other public health professionals, reporting and compliance systems related to laws, regulations, and policies.

- Monitors reporting and compliance systems for quality and appropriate use of resources.

- Analyzes data from reporting and compliance systems.

- Develops reports for public health officials and other decision-makers as required by laws, regulations, and policies.

- Participates in coordinating emergency preparedness and response efforts, including receipt and use of the Strategic National Stockpile.

STANDARD 6. EVALUATION
The public health nurse evaluates the health status of the population.

Measurement Criteria:

The public health nurse:

- Participates in a systematic, ongoing, and criterion-based evaluation of service outcomes with the population and other stakeholders.

- Collects data systematically, applying epidemiological and scientific methods to determine the effectiveness of public health nursing interventions on policies, programs, and services.

- Participates in process and outcome evaluation by monitoring activities in programs or services.

- Applies ongoing assessment data to revise plans, interventions, and activities, as appropriate.

- Documents the results of the evaluation including changes or recommendations to enhance effectiveness of interventions.

- Disseminates the process and outcome evaluation results to the population and other stakeholders in accordance with state and federal laws and regulations, as appropriate.

Additional Measurement Criteria for the Advanced Practice Public Health Nurse:

The advanced practice public health nurse:

- Designs an evaluation plan with other public health experts, and with representatives from the population and from stakeholders.

- Modifies the evaluation plan for policies, programs, or services, as appropriate.

- Evaluates the effectiveness of the plan in relationship to expected and unexpected outcomes.

- Synthesizes the results of the evaluation analyses to determine the effect of the plan on populations, organizations, and other stakeholder groups.

- Applies the results of the evaluation analyses to recommend or make process or outcomes changes in policies, programs, or services, as appropriate.

Standards of Professional Performance

Standard 7. Quality of Practice
The public health nurse systematically enhances the quality and effectiveness of nursing practice.

Measurement Criteria:

The public health nurse:

- Demonstrates quality through the application of the nursing process in a responsible, accountable, and ethical manner.

- Implements new knowledge and performance improvement activities to initiate changes in public health nursing practice and in the delivery of care to populations.

- Incorporates creativity and innovation in activities to improve the quality of nursing practice.

- Participates in the development, implementation, and evaluation of procedures and guidelines to improve the quality of practice.

- Participates in the scope of the performance improvement activities as appropriate to the nurse's position, education, and practice environment. Such activities may include:

  - Identifying aspects of practice important for quality monitoring.

  - Employing evidence-based indicators to monitor the quality and effectiveness of nursing practice.

  - Collecting data to monitor public health nursing practice, including availability, accessibility, acceptability, quality, and effectiveness of policies, programs, and services.

  - Monitoring indicators of quality and effectiveness of policies, programs, and services.

  - Analyzing the data to identify opportunities for improving nursing practice.

  - Formulating recommendations to improve nursing practice or outcomes.

Continued ▶

- Implementing activities to enhance the quality of nursing practice.
- Participating with the population and other professionals, organizations, and stakeholders in the evaluation of policies, programs, and services.
- Assessing professional performance factors related to population safety, accessibility to services, program effectiveness, and cost–benefit options.
- Analyzing organization and program processes and systems to remove or decrease barriers and to enhance assets.

- Documents the delivery of programs and services in ways that reflect the quality measures.
- Obtains and maintains professional certification, if available, in the area of expertise.

Additional Measurement Criteria for the Advanced Practice Public Health Nurse:

The advanced practice public health nurse:

- Designs performance improvement initiatives related to policies, programs, and services based on existing evidence.
- Implements initiatives to evaluate the need for change.
- Evaluates the practice environment and quality of nursing care rendered in relation to existing evidence-based information.
- Identifies opportunities for the generation and use of research to enhance the evidence base for public health nursing practice.

STANDARD 8. EDUCATION
The public health nurse attains knowledge and competency that reflects current nursing and public health practice.

Measurement Criteria:

The public health nurse:

- Participates in ongoing educational activities to maintain and enhance the knowledge and skills necessary to promote the health of the population.

- Seeks experiences to develop and maintain competence in the skills needed to implement policies, programs, and services for populations.

- Identifies learning needs based on nursing and public health knowledge, the various roles the nurse may assume, and the changing needs of the population.

- Identifies changes in the statutory requirements for the practice of nursing and public health.

- Maintains professional records that provide evidence of competency and lifelong learning.

- Seeks experiences and formal and independent learning activities to maintain and develop clinical and professional skills and knowledge.

Additional Measurement Criteria for the Advanced Practice Public Health Nurse:

The advanced practice public health nurse:

- Uses current research findings and other evidence to expand nursing and public health knowledge, enhance role performance, and increase knowledge of professional issues.

STANDARD 9. PROFESSIONAL PRACTICE EVALUATION

The public health nurse evaluates one's own nursing practice in relation to professional practice standards and guidelines, relevant statutes, rules, and regulations.

Measurement Criteria:

The public health nurse:

- Implements age-appropriate population-focused policies, programs, and services in a culturally and ethnically sensitive manner.

- Engages in self-evaluation of practice on a regular basis, identifying areas of strength as well as areas in which professional development would be beneficial.

- Seeks feedback regarding one's own practice from community and professional partners and other peers.

- Implements plans for accomplishing goals in one's own work plan.

- Integrates the knowledge of current practice standards, guidelines, statutes, rules, and regulations into one's own work plans.

- Provides rationale for professional practice beliefs, decisions, and actions as part of the evaluation process.

- Applies knowledge of current practice standards, guidelines, statutes, certification, and regulation in self-evaluation and peer review.

Additional Measurement Criteria for the Advanced Practice Public Health Nurse:

The advanced practice public health nurse:

- Engages in a formal systematic process seeking feedback regarding one's own practice from peers, professional colleagues, community and professional organizations, and stakeholders.

- Analyzes practice in relation to advanced certification requirements as appropriate.

STANDARD 10. COLLEGIALITY AND PROFESSIONAL RELATIONSHIPS

The public health nurse establishes collegial partnerships while interacting with representatives of the population, organizations, and health and human services professionals, and contributes to the professional development of peers, students, colleagues, and others.

Measurement Criteria:

The public health nurse:

- Shares knowledge and skills with peers, students, colleagues, and others.

- Interacts with peers, students, colleagues, and others to enhance professional nursing or public health practice and role performance of self and others.

- Mentors other public health nurses, colleagues, students, and others as appropriate.

- Maintains compassionate and caring relationships with professional colleagues and other stakeholders involved in population health.

- Contributes to an environment that fosters ongoing educational experiences for colleagues, healthcare professionals, and the population.

- Contributes to a supportive, healthy, and safe work environment.

Additional Measurement Criteria for the Advanced Practice Public Health Nurse:

The advanced practice public health nurse:

- Models expert practice to multi-sector team members and the population.

- Designs mentoring policies and programs for public health nurses and other colleagues.

- Participates in activities that contribute to the development of the advanced practice nursing role in public health.

STANDARD 11. COLLABORATION

The public health nurse collaborates with representatives of the population, organizations, and health and human service professionals in providing for and promoting the health of the population.

Measurement Criteria:

The public health nurse:

- Communicates with various constituencies in the community to gather information and develop partnerships and coalitions to address population-focused health concerns.

- Partners with individuals, groups, and community-based organizations in the assessment, planning, implementing, and evaluation of population-focused policies, programs, and services.

- Articulates nursing and public health knowledge and skills to the interdisciplinary team, administrators, policy makers, and other multi-sector partners.

- Partners with other disciplines in teaching, program development and implementation, evaluation, research, and public policy advocacy.

- Contributes to the multi-sector team in implementing public health regulatory requirements such as case identification, program management, and mandatory reporting.

- Partners with key individuals, groups, coalitions, and organizations to effect change in public health policies, programs, and services to generate positive outcomes.

- Documents collaborative interactions and processes related to policies, programs, and services.

Additional Measurement Criteria for the Advanced Practice Public Health Nurse:

The advanced practice public health nurse:

- Develops alliances and coalitions with community organizations to address public health policies, programs, and services.

- Initiates collaborative efforts across constituencies in the population.

- Designs educational, administrative, research, and public policy programs to promote the health of the population.

- Develops systems for documentation and accountability in nursing and public health nursing practice, including compliance with regulatory requirements.

STANDARD 12. ETHICS

The public health nurse integrates ethical provisions in all areas of practice.

Measurement Criteria:

The public health nurse:

- Applies *Code of Ethics for Nurses with Interpretive Statements* (ANA, 2001) and *Principles of the Ethical Practice of Public Health* (Public Health Leadership Society, 2002) to guide public health nursing practice.

- Delivers programs and services in a manner that preserves, protects, and promotes the autonomy, dignity, and rights of the population or community as well as individuals.

- Applies ethical standards in advocating for health and social policy.

- Maintains individual confidentiality within legal and regulatory parameters.

- Assists populations, communities, and individuals in developing skills for self-advocacy.

- Maintains professional relationships and boundaries with individuals and groups within the population while delivering public health services and programs.

- Demonstrates a commitment to fostering an environment and conditions in which healthy lifestyles may be practiced by self, colleagues, and identified populations.

- Contributes to resolving social and environmental issues and barriers to healthy living conditions.

- Contributes to resolving ethical issues involving colleagues, community groups, systems, and other stakeholders.

- Reports activities that are illegal, inconsistent with accepted standards of practice, or reflective of impaired practice.

Additional Measurement Criteria for the Advanced Practice Public Health Nurse:

The advanced practice public health nurse:

- Informs populations and communities of the risks, benefits, and outcomes of policies, programs, and services.

- Informs administrators or others of the risks, benefits, and outcomes of policies, programs, and services, and related decisions that affect the delivery of health-related services.

- Partners with multi-sector teams to address ethical risks, benefits, and outcomes of policies, programs, and services.

- Promotes solutions to social and environmental issues and barriers to healthy living conditions.

STANDARD 13. RESEARCH
The public health nurse integrates research findings into practice.

Measurement Criteria:

The public health nurse:

- Utilizes the best available evidence, including research findings, to guide practice, policy, and service delivery decisions.

- Actively participates in research activities at various levels appropriate to one's own level of education and position. Such activities may include:

  - Identifying community and professional opportunities suitable for nursing and public health research.

  - Participating in data collection.

  - Participating in agency-, organization-, or population-focused research committees or programs.

  - Sharing research activities and findings with peers and others.

  - Implementing research protocols.

  - Critically analyzing and interpreting research for application to population-focused practice.

  - Applying nursing and public health research findings in the development of policies, programs, and services for populations.

  - Incorporating research as a basis for learning.

- Actively involves communities, populations, organizations, and other stakeholder groups in a participatory research process.

Additional Measurement Criteria for the Advanced Practice Public Health Nurse:

The advanced practice public health nurse:

- Contributes to nursing knowledge by conducting or synthesizing research that discovers, examines, and evaluates knowledge, theories, models, criteria, and creative approaches to improve healthcare practice and outcomes.

- Formally disseminates research findings through consultation, presentations, publications, and the use of other media.

STANDARD 14. RESOURCE UTILIZATION

The public health nurse considers factors related to safety, effectiveness, cost, and impact on practice and on the population in the planning and delivery of nursing and public health programs, policies, and services.

Measurement Criteria:

The public health nurse:

- Evaluates factors such as safety, effectiveness, availability, cost and benefits, efficiencies, and impact on practice and on the population, when choosing practice options that would result in the same expected outcome.

- Assists representatives of specific populations and other stakeholders in identifying and securing appropriate and available services to address health-related needs.

- Assigns or delegates tasks taking into consideration the concerns of the population, potential for harm, complexity of the task, and predictability of the outcomes.

- Helps the population to become informed about the options, costs, risks, and benefits of policies, programs, and services.

Additional Measurement Criteria for the Advanced Practice Public Health Nurse:

The advanced practice public health nurse:

- Utilizes organizational and community resources to formulate multi-sector plans for policies, programs, and services.

- Develops innovative approaches to community and public health concerns that include effective resource utilization and improvement of quality.

- Develops evaluation strategies to demonstrate cost effectiveness and efficiency factors associated with nursing and public health practice and outcomes.

STANDARD 15. LEADERSHIP

The public health nurse provides leadership in nursing and public health.

Measurement Criteria:

The public health nurse:

- Engages in multi-sector team development and coalition building, including other professionals, the population, and stakeholders.

- Promotes healthy community and work environments at local, regional, national, and international levels.

- Articulates the mission, goals, action plan, and outcome measures of nursing and public health programs and services to other professionals and the population.

- Advocates for opportunities for continuous, lifelong learning for self and others.

- Teaches peers, stakeholders, and others in the population to succeed through mentoring and other strategies.

- Exhibits creativity and flexibility through times of change.

- Fosters a culture where systems are monitored and evaluated to improve the quality of policies, programs, and services for populations.

- Coordinates programs and services across various community settings and among the multi-sector team.

- Serves in leadership roles in the work setting, in the community, and with the population.

- Promotes advancement of public health and nursing through participation in professional organizations.

- Functions as a public health team leader in emergency preparedness and response situations, delegating tasks as delineated in standardized protocols.

Additional Measurement Criteria for the Advanced Practice Public Health Nurse:

The advanced practice public health nurse:

- Advocates with decision-makers to influence public health policies, programs, and services to promote healthy populations.

- Provides direction to enhance the effectiveness of policies, programs, and services provided by the multi-sector team.

- Initiates and revises protocols or guidelines to reflect evidence-based practice, to reflect accepted changes in program and service delivery, or to address emerging problems in the population.

- Promotes communication of information and advancement of nursing and public health through writing, publishing, and presentations for professional or lay audiences.

- Demonstrates innovative approaches to public health and nursing practice to improve health outcomes for populations.

- Organizes formal plans in response to public health emergencies for populations.

STANDARD 16. ADVOCACY

The public health nurse advocates to protect the health, safety, and rights of the population.

Measurement Criteria:

The public health nurse:

- Incorporates the identified needs of the population in policy development and program or service planning.

- Integrates advocacy into the implementation of policies, programs, and services for the population.

- Evaluates the effectiveness of advocating for the population when assessing the expected outcomes.

- Includes confidentiality, ethical, legal, privacy, and professional guidelines in policy development and other issues.

- Demonstrates skill in advocating before providers and stakeholders on behalf of the population.

- Strives to resolve conflicting expectations from populations, providers, and other stakeholders to ensure the safety and to guard the best interest of the population and to preserve the professional integrity of the nurse.

Additional Measurement Criteria for the Advanced Practice Public Health Nurse:

The advanced practice public health nurse:

- Demonstrates skill in advocating before public representatives and decision-makers on behalf of the populations, programs, and services.

- Designs materials for the advocacy process that are based on the needs of the populations, programs, and services.

- Exhibits fiscal responsibility and integrity in the policy development process.

- Serves as an expert for peers, populations, providers, and other stakeholders in promoting and implementing public health policies.

GLOSSARY

Advocacy. The act of pleading or arguing in favor of a cause, idea, or policy on someone else's behalf, with the object of developing the community, system, individual, or family's capacity to plead their own cause or act on their own behalf.

Assessment. The regular and systematic collection, analysis, and dissemination of information on the health of the community or population, including statistics on health status, community health needs, and epidemiological and other studies of health problems.

Assurance. Assuring that services necessary to achieve agreed-upon goals are provided by encouraging actions by other entities (private or public), by requiring such action through regulation, or by providing services directly.

Coalition building. The process by which parties (individuals, organizations, or groups) come together to form a temporary alliance or union to work together for a common purpose and to enhance each other's capacity for mutual benefit and common purpose.

Collaboration. Work with another person or group to achieve some end.

Community. A set of persons in interaction, being and experiencing together, who may or may not share a sense of place or belonging, and who act intentionally for a common purpose. A community is different from the group of people who constitute it and can interact with other entities as a unit.

Community-based organizations. Private nonprofit organizations or other types of groups that work within a community for the improvement of some aspect of that community.

Cultural competence. A set of congruent behaviors, attitudes, and policies that come together in a system or agency or among professionals and enable the system, agency, or professionals to work effectively in cross-cultural settings.

Cultural diversity. The coexistence of different ethnic, gender, racial, and socioeconomic groups.

Determinants of health. Social, economic, and healthcare factors that affect health and well-being independently or in conjunction with each other at the population or community level. Comprehensive factors involve relevant social, economic, environmental, behavioral, political, health, and healthcare indicators that describe the essential features of a social structure and system and the processes through which change occurs.

Ecological model. A model of health that emphasizes the linkages and relationships among multiple factors (or determinants) affecting health.

Environmental health. Those aspects of human health, including quality of life, that are determined by physical, chemical, biological, social, and psychological processes in the environment. It also refers to the theory and practice of assessing, correcting, controlling, or preventing those factors in the environment that can adversely affect the health of the present and future generations.

Epidemiology. The study of the distribution of determinants and antecedents of health and disease in human populations. The ultimate goal is to identify the underlying causes of a disease and then to apply those findings to disease prevention and health promotion.

Evidence. Verifiable knowledge on which belief is based.

Evidence-based practice. An approach to public healthcare practice in which the public health nurse is aware of the evidence in support of one's clinical practice, and the strength of that evidence.

Health status (of a population). The level of illness or wellness of a population at a designated time.

Interdisciplinary team. A group of individuals who rely on each other's overlapping skills and discipline-based knowledge to achieve synergistic effects where outcomes are enhanced and more comprehensive than the simple aggregation of individual members' efforts.

Multi-sector team. A partnership of community organizations and groups representing a variety of viewpoints and perspectives which impact public health issues.

Outcomes. Long-term objectives that define optimal, measurable future levels of health status, maximum acceptable levels of disease, injury, or dysfunction, or prevalence of risk factors.

Partnership. A relationship in which two or more people or groups operate together to achieve a common goal.

Performance improvement. A process that considers the organizational context, describes desired performance, identifies gaps between desired and actual performance, identifies root causes, selects interventions to close the gaps, and measures changes in performance with the goal of achieving desired results or outcomes.

Policy development. Applying comprehensive public health scientific knowledge for decision-making. Policy development includes a systematic course of action to establish priorities, determine effective strategies and interventions, and use community resources, including regulation and law, to achieve the community's goals.

Population. Those living in a specific geographic area (e.g., a neighborhood, community, city, or county) or those in a particular group (e.g., racial, ethnic, age) who experience a disproportionate burden of poor health outcomes.

Population-focused. An approach to health care that operates at the population level of the ecological model.

Priorities. A ranking or ordering of diagnoses, strategies, or activities that identifies those that are most important or that should be addressed first.

Social justice. The principle that all persons are entitled to have their basic human needs met, regardless of differences in economic status, class, gender, race, ethnicity, citizenship, religion, age, sexual orientation, disability, or health. This includes the eradication of poverty and illiteracy, the establishment of sound environmental policy, and equality of opportunity for healthy personal and social development.

Stakeholder. A person or organization that has a legitimate interest in what a public health entity does.

Standard. An authoritative statement, defined and promoted by the profession, by which the quality of practice, service, or education can be evaluated.

Strategic National Stockpile. Large quantities of medicines, antidotes, and medical supples needed to respond to a wide range of circumstances where supplies of critical medical items in any jurisdiction would be rapidly depleted; the stockpile is managed by the Centers for Disease Control and Prevention (CDC).

Surveillance. The systematic collection, analysis, interpretation, and dissemination of data to assist in the planning, implementation, and evaluation of public health interventions and programs.

References

American Nurses Association (ANA). (1973). *Standards of nursing practice.* Washington, DC: American Nurses Publishing. (Also available as appendix in ANA 2004a.)

American Nurses Association (ANA). (1986). *Standards of community nursing practice.* Washington, DC: American Nurses Publishing.

American Nurses Association (ANA). (1999). *Scope and standards of public health nursing.* Washington, DC: American Nurses Publishing.

American Nurses Association (ANA). (2001). *Code of ethics for nurses with interpretive statements.* Washington, DC: American Nurses Publishing.

American Nurses Association (ANA). (2003). *Nursing's social policy statement, 2nd edition.* Washington, DC: Nursesbooks.org.

American Nurses Association (ANA). (2004a). *Nursing: Scope and standards of practice.* Silver Spring, MD: Nursesbooks.org.

American Nurses Association (ANA). (2004b). *Scope and standards for nurse administrators, 2nd edition.* Silver Spring, MD: Nursesbooks.org.

American Public Health Association (APHA). Public Health Nursing Section (PHNS). (1996). The definition and role of public health nursing. Retrieved August 23, 2005, from http://www.csuchico.edu/~horst/about/definition.html.

American Public Health Association (APHA). Public Health Nursing Section (PHNS). (2006). *Environmental health principles and recommendations for public health nursing.* Washington, DC: APHA

Association of Community Health Nursing Educators (ACHNE). (2000). *Essentials of baccalaureate nursing education for entry level community health nursing practice.* Latham, NY: ACHNE.

Association of Community Health Nursing Educators (ACHNE). (2003). *Essentials of master's level nursing education for advanced community/ public health nursing practice.* Latham, NY: ACHNE.

Centers for Disease Control and Prevention (CDC). (2001). *National public health performance standards.* Retrieved August 23, 2005, from http://www.cdc.gov/od/ocphp/nphpsp/TheInstruments.htm.

Council on Linkages Between Academia and Public Health Practice. (2001). *Core competencies for public health professionals.* Retrieved August 23, 2005, from http://www.phf.org/competencies.htm.

Department of Health and Human Services (HHS). (2000). *Healthy people 2010, 2nd edition.* Washington, DC: U.S. Government Printing Office.

Institute of Medicine (IOM). (1988). *The future of public health.* Washington, DC: National Academy Press.

Institute of Medicine (IOM). (1995). *Nursing, health, and the environment.* Washington, DC: National Academy Press.

Institute of Medicine (IOM). (2003a). *The future of the public's health in the twenty-first century.* Washington, DC: National Academy Press.

Institute of Medicine (IOM). (2003b). *Who will keep the public healthy?* Washington, DC: National Academy Press.

Public Health Leadership Society. (2002). *Principles of the ethical practice of public health, version 2.2.* Retrieved August 23, 2005, from http://www.phls.org.

Quad Council of Public Health Nursing Organizations. (2004). Public health nursing competencies. *Public Health Nursing, 21*(5), 443–452.

Quad Council of Public Health Nursing Organizations & American Nurses Association. (1999). *Scope and standards of public health nursing practice.* Washington, DC: American Nurses Publishing.

Tickner, J. (2002). Precaution and preventive public health policy. *Policy Health Reports, 117*, 493–497.

Tickner, J., & Raffensberger, C. (1998). *The precautionary principle in action: A handbook, 1st edition*. Retrieved August 16, 2006, from http://www.sehn.org/rtfdocs/handbook-rtf.rtf.

Appendix A
Comparison of Multiple Determinants of Population Health Using an Ecological Framework and Selected Public Health Nursing Intervention Models

An ecological framework for guiding public health nursing interventions considers multiple determinants of population health (individual behavior; social, family, and community networks of support; living and working conditions; and policies) in conjunction with the levels of potential influence (macro-upstream, midlevel, micro-downstream, and proximate) on those determinants.

References

ASTDN Model
Association of State and Territorial Directors of Nursing (ASTDN) and American Nurses Association (ANA). (2000). *Public health nursing: A partner for healthy populations.* Washington, D.C.: American Nurses Publishing.

EPI Model
Koepsell, T.D., & N. S. Weiss. (2003). *Diseases and populations in epidemiologic methods*, pp. 17–36. New York: Oxford University Press.

Laffrey and Kulbok Model
Laffrey, S.C., & P. A. Kulbok. (1999). An integrative model for holistic community health nursing. *Journal of Holistic Nursing 17* (1): 88–103.

MN Model
Keller, L.O., S. Strohschein, B. Lia-Hoagberg, & M.A. Schaffer. (2004).Population-based public health interventions: Practice-based and evidence supported. *Public Health Nursing 21*(5): 453–468. (September).

Salmon Model
Salmon, M.E. (1993). Public health nursing, The opportunity of a lifetime. *American Journal of Public Health 83*(1): 674–675.

Determinant Category Intervention Model	Individual	Social, Family, And Community	Living And Working Conditions	Broad Social, Economic, Cultural, Health, Environmental Conditions and Policies
Anderson/Mcfarlane Model Community as Partner	Communities are composed of individuals, who are considered as equal partners with the nurse in this model. The community's people are at the core of the model.	The model begins with a community assessment wheel, considering the core (demography, values, beliefs, and history) and eight subsystem components, of which health and social services is one. Communities have a normal line of defense (health); a flexible line of defense (buffer zone); and a line of resistance. The degree of reaction to stressors becomes part of the nursing diagnosis.	Components of the subsystems of a community include the physical environment, safety and transportation, communication, economics, and recreation. Living and working conditions are considered across more than one of these subsystems as defined in this model.	The healthy community functions in equilibrium within its normal line of defense. Dis-equilibrium occurs when internal or external stressors (temporary or permanent) are introduced. The community responds to stressors based on its previous patterns of coping and problem-solving capabilities, in the context of this model.
ASTDN Model (Association of State and Territorial Directors of Nursing)	Care of the individual provides a foundation for population health practice through the application of knowledge to the aggregate.	Families and communities are served through fluid activity between nursing practice (critical thinking, the nursing process, a holistic approach) and the Core Public Health Functions and Essential Services.	The nurse acts on conditions in the environment through critical thinking and the nursing process by performing the duties of the Essential Public Health Services.	The practice of nursing and the Core Public Health Functions provide a framework for organizing, delivering, and evaluating interventions aimed at improving health with the Essential Public Health Services further delineating the functions.
EPI Model	**Multifactoral human—environment interaction:** Individual effects are influenced by varying emphasis of individual (genetics, biology) and environmental (physical, social, biological) factors.	Existing biological and genetic factors in a family or community interact with social, physical, and biological factors in the environment to determine health outcomes.	**Multiple ecological interactions:** The health impact of biological, social, and physical factors in the environment varies by the public health problem or disease under consideration.	**Multiple ecological interactions:** Social, physical, and biological manipulation of the environment affect health. Measures for controlling disease or improving health can be evaluated in terms of the total effect on the ecosystem and human health.

Model				
Laffrey & Kulbok (1999), *Integrative Model For Community Health Promotion*	**Multidimensional Client Systems:** Individual most delimited level. **Focus of Care (across all client systems):** Health Promotion, Illness Prevention, and Illness Care. The goal of C/PHN is a healthy community, achieved through health promotion interventions. No matter where C/PHN care begins, it ultimately leads to health promotion of the community.	**Client System:** Family, aggregate, and community.	Each successive client system or level provides the environment for the preceding level. Family, aggregate, and community compose the environment for the individual level; aggregate and community make up the environment for the family, and the community is the environment for the aggregate. Different kinds of assessments and nursing interventions are appropriate at each level of client within the system.	**Client System:** Increasingly complex from delimited individual system to complex community and society. C/PHN is holistic in nature and is population-focused in that it addresses multiple levels of client and multiple levels of care within the total system.
MN Model *PHN Interventions*	Three levels of practice are defined in the population-based model. Interventions at the individual level focus on changing attitudes, knowledge, beliefs, practices, and behaviors. These interventions contribute to the overall goal of improving population health. Interventions of particular relevance to this level of practice include referral, case management, health teaching, counseling, and consultation.	Population-based community practice changes community norms, community attitudes, community awareness, practices, and behaviors. Interventions that may have particular relevance at this level include collaboration, coalition building, and community organizing. In addition, surveillance and screening are particularly critical to maintaining health in a community.	Population-based community practice is concerned with the environment of individuals, families, and communities. Interventions that may also have particular relevance at this level include collaboration, coalition building, and community organizing.	Population systems-focused practice changes organizations, policies, laws, and power structure. The focus of practice is on systems that affect health. Interventions that may be particularly relevant to this practice include advocacy, social marketing, and policy development, as well as collaboration and organizing.
Salmon Model	The individual is the point at which the continuum of intervention by the public health nurse begins. There are human and biological determinants of health which affect the individual's contribution to the health status continuum. The public health nurse must understand and consider these as one element of the construct for practice.	Social determinants of health are a category of focus in this model. Valuing of the public good lies at the ethical core of this model. The public health nurse considers interventions that affect social and political processes, with prevention being the primary focus.	Environmental determinants of health are one of the four categories of factors affecting the health of the public which the public health nurse considers in carrying out the nursing process. Environmental factors, like the other three determinants, are considered at individual, group, community, family, and population levels.	This model describes medical, technological, and organizational determinants of health as the fourth category. This category considers the organization of the total healthcare system. Public health nursing interventions are targeted and intentional, based on consideration of all four aspects of the construct.

APPENDIX B. *STANDARDS OF COMMUNITY HEALTH NURSING PRACTICE* (1986)

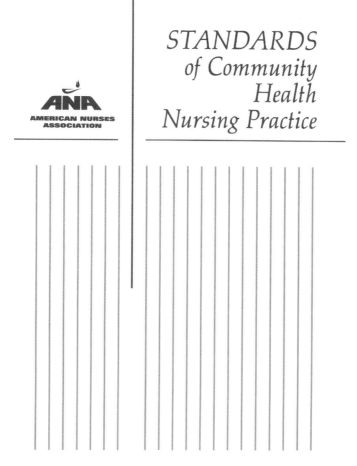

STANDARDS
of Community
Health
Nursing Practice

AMERICAN NURSES
ASSOCIATION

STANDARDS
of Community Health
Nursing Practice

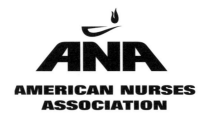

ANA

AMERICAN NURSES
ASSOCIATION

CONTENTS

INTRODUCTION

The purpose of *Standards of Community Health Nursing Practice* is to fulfill the profession's obligation to provide a means of improving the quality of care. Standards reflect the current state of knowledge in the field and are therefore provisional, dynamic, and subject to testing and subsequent change. Representing agreed-upon levels of practice, standards are developed to characterize, to measure, and to provide guidance in achieving excellence in care.[1] The standards developed by the American Nurses Association for various specialty areas or fields of interest within nursing are based on the generic *Standards of Nursing Practice*, published by ANA in 1973.[2]

The community health standards presented here are a revision of *Standards of Community Health Nursing Practice* developed in 1973 by the Division on Community Health Nursing Practice (now the Council of Community Health Nurses).[3] These revised standards apply to any setting in which community health nursing is practiced, involving care of communities, families, and individuals. These standards apply both to generalists and specialists in community health nursing practice. These standards were written within the framework of the nursing process, which includes data collection, diagnosis, planning, treatment, and evaluation.[4]

This document gives the rationale and criteria for each standard. The criteria, divided into structure, process, and outcome criteria, provide a means by which attainment of the standard may be specifically measured; however, the criteria for each standard are not exhaustive. Within appropriate standards, the process criteria have been further divided into nurse generalist and nurse specialist activities related to the community, family, and individual.

Standards of Community Health Nursing Practice should be used in conjunction with the following ANA publications: *Nursing: A Social Policy Statement,*[5] *Standards of Nursing Practice,*[6] *Code for Nurses with Interpretive Statements,*[7] *A Conceptual Model of Community Health Nursing,*[8] *A Guide for Community-Based Nursing Services,*[9] *The Scope of Practice of the Primary Health Care Nurse Practitioner,*[10] and *Community-Based Nursing Services: Innovative Models.*[11]

Various standards in this document have criteria that address professional performance, such as use of theory, professional development, interdisciplinary collaboration, and research. Implicit throughout the standards are the nurse's accountability to the client, respect for the client's rights, and advocacy for the client.

The rest of this Introduction to *Standards of Community Health Nursing Practice* provides a definition of the practice area, discusses ethical responsibilities, and presents guidelines for using the standards.

Definition of the Practice Area

Community health nursing practice promotes and preserves the health of populations by integrating the skills and knowledge relevant to both nursing and public health. The practice is comprehensive and general, and is not limited to a particular age or diagnostic group; it is continual, and is not limited to episodic care. In this document, the terms *community health nursing* and *public health nursing* are synonymous (see the Glossary).

Community health nursing practice promotes the public's health. The programs, services, and institutions involved in public health emphasize promotion and maintenance of the population's health, and the prevention and limitation of disease. Public health activities change with changing technology and social values, but the goals remain the same: to reduce the amount of disease, premature death, discomfort, and disability.[12]

While community health nursing practice includes nursing directed to individuals, families, and groups, the dominant responsibility is to the population as a whole. Nurses' efforts to promote and maintain the population's health entail the understanding and application of (a) concepts of public health and community; (b) skills of community organization and development; and (c) nursing care of selected individuals, families, and groups for health promotion, health maintenance, health education, and coordination of care.

As noted in the Glossary, the World Health Organization defines a *community* as a social group determined by geographical boundaries and/or common values and interests. Its members interact with each other. It functions within a particular social structure, exhibits and creates norms and values, and establishes social institutions.[13]

The nurse's actions reflect awareness of the need for comprehensive health planning in partnership with communities; the influence of social, economic, ecological, and political issues; the needs of populations at risk; and the dynamic forces that stimulate change. Because the nurse's primary responsibility is to a population, some practice occurs through organization and coordination of the actions of others in response to health needs. When care is given to individuals, families, or groups, this responsibility dictates that the nurse's priorities concerning which clients to serve are determined by the needs of the population.

Professional community health nurses recognize that many local health issues are directly and profoundly affected by larger policy issues. Consequently, their practice reflects awareness of and responsiveness to legislative action and other means by which health and social policies are set at all levels within the health care system and the government.

The theoretical and factual context within which the community health nurse understands phenomena and their interrelationships derives from an interdisciplinary base including public health, the humanities, the social and behavioral sciences, epidemiology, and nursing science.

Community health nursing practice should be consistent with the World Health Organization's concept of primary health care as "essential health care made universally accessible to individuals and families in the community by means acceptable to them, through their full participation, and at a cost that the community and country can afford. Primary health care forms an integral part both of the country's health system (of which it is the nucleus) and of the overall social and economic development of the community."[14] Imbedded in this definition is the assumption that health care is a right and not a privilege.

Appendix B: Standards of Community Health Nursing Practice   **57**

Ethical Responsibilities

The Council of Community Health Nurses accepts the ethical standards made explicit in the *Code for Nurses with Interpretive Statements.* Nurses who work in the community may encounter many situations in which human rights and freedoms are in jeopardy. Assuming that health care is a right, community health nurses have the responsibility to advocate for individuals and families, to identify and rectify gaps in health care services, and to influence health and social policies that are inconsistent with this basic right.

Communities, families, and individuals have the right to a clear explanation of proposed health care, due consideration of their wishes, and an opportunity to ask questions prior to making decisions about care. The rights of the individual client include the right to be autonomous, the right to make an informed decision, and the right to one's domain, including one's body, life, property, and privacy. Competent clients have the right to deny access to their home and the right not to seek or follow health care recommendations. However, if the individual or group poses a specific health risk to the public, certain rights may be forfeited for the protection of the community.

When the client is a child or an adult whose competence is questionable, an evaluation must be made of the client's or the care-giver's ability to make informed decisions about care. In the case of the infant or the very young child, the parent(s) or guardian(s) should make informed decisions about care, provided the child's rights are not violated. Conflicts will arise between rights of individuals and rights of families—for example, in cases of domestic violence or neglect—and between rights of individuals and the public's right to protection. In such instances, the community health nurse should seek legal and/or ethical consultation to determine the best course of action.

Community leaders, organizations, and residents with whom the community health nurse collaborates have the right to judicious protection of privileged information they share with the nurse. They also have the right to choose not to participate in the development of community health programs. Communities have the right and responsibility to identify their own health needs and to negotiate with the community health nurse regarding priorities for intervention and program development. The community health nurse, in turn, has the responsibility to provide information or assist with the collection and interpretation of information necessary to this process.

Guidelines for Using the Standards

These standards apply broadly to community health nursing and as such apply to subspecialty areas of community health nursing, including home health, occupational health, and school health, and to primary health care nurse practitioners functioning in these and other specialty areas. These standards are to be used in conjunction with standards of practice of the subspecialties for which standards have been developed.

These standards reflect two practice levels: that of the generalist prepared at the baccalaureate level, and that of the specialist prepared at the graduate level.

In the absence of the specialist, the generalist assumes many aspects of the comprehensive role of the specialist. These standards outline levels of professional nursing practice to be achieved by the nurse. Nurses prepared at less than the baccalaureate level are not educationally prepared to meet these standards, but may use them as a guide in providing care and pursuing their own professional development.

The community health nurse generalist, prepared in nursing at the baccalaureate level, provides care primarily to individuals, families, and groups in a wide range of primary care settings with an understanding of the values and concepts of population-based practice. The generalist participates in implementation of community-wide assessment and in the planning, implementation, and evaluation of health programs and services. The generalist draws on the expertise of the specialist. If a specialist is not available in the practice setting, the use of a consultant is advisable.

The master's-prepared or doctorally prepared community health nurse specialist can and may perform all functions of the generalist. In addition, the specialist possesses substantial clinical experience with families and groups; expertise in the formulation of health and social policy and the assessment of the health of a community or population; and proficiency in planning, implementation, and evaluation of population-focused programs. These skills are based on knowledge of epidemiology, demography, biometrics, community structure and organization, community development, management, program evaluation, and policy development. The community health nurse specialist also engages in research, theory testing, and theory development relevant to community practice and health policy development. While there are master's-prepared nurses whose area of expertise is the care of a particular segment of the community (for example, persons at a given age level or in a particular setting in the community), the preparation of the community health nurse specialist described in this document emphasizes skills to promote the health of an entire community.

This document has been developed to help nurses in practice to validate the quality of care and to improve care. Validation of care is derived from documentation that is concise, standardized, timely, and retrievable. These standards should be used in systems of quality assurance to evaluate nursing services and to institute programs of peer review. These standards should be made specific to the practice setting and can be used to develop assessment tools and formats for planning and recording care. The content for community health certification examinations should be derived from these standards.

STANDARDS

Standard I. Theory

THE NURSE APPLIES THEORETICAL CONCEPTS AS A BASIS FOR DECISIONS IN PRACTICE.

Rationale

Theoretical concepts define the context within which the community health nurse understands phenomena and their interrelationships, thereby providing a framework for assessment, intervention, and evaluation. Through the application of theoretical concepts in practice, the nurse generates questions for investigation. Theoretical concepts for community health nursing are derived from intradisciplinary and interdisciplinary sources, including nursing, public health, social and behavioral sciences, and physical sciences.

Structure Criteria

1. Resource materials discussing the conceptual bases for practice are accessible.
2. Theory-related professional development programs are accessible.
3. Theory-based nursing actions are documented within the practice setting and are congruent with agency philosophy.

Process Criteria

The nurse—

1. examines personal and professional assumptions about community health practice.
2. considers alternative theoretical concepts.
3. uses theoretical concepts and critical thinking in practice—
   a. to identify patterns and incongruencies.
   b. to generate and test hypotheses.
4. Shares and interprets theoretical information with colleagues, individuals, families, and the community.

Outcome Criterion

Theory-based nursing actions are used, tested, and evaluated within the practice setting.

Standard II. Data Collection

THE NURSE SYSTEMATICALLY COLLECTS DATA THAT ARE COMPREHENSIVE AND ACCURATE.

Rationale

Data collection is essential to a realistic assessment of the community, family, and individual. The process must be comprehensive, accurate, systematic, and continual to allow the community health nurse to reach sound conclusions and plan for appropriate interventions.

Structure Criteria

1. A data collection method is used in the setting; the method provides for—
   a. systematic and complete collection of data.
   b. frequent updating of records.
   c. retrievability of data from the record-keeping system.
   d. confidentiality when appropriate.
2. The practice setting allows access to data on the community, family, and individual.
3. A record-keeping system based on the nursing process is used in the setting; the system provides for concise, comprehensive, accurate, and continual recording.
4. The practice setting has in place a logical system of data collection and retrieval that allows priorities to be set for service to communities, families, and individuals.

Process Criteria

COMMUNITY

The nurse generalist—
1. in collaboration with the specialist and in partnership with the community, collects community data, including but not limited to community resources, power structures, vital statistics, demographics, community dynamics, and socioeconomic, cultural, and environmental characteristics.
2. uses data sources such as legal documents, vital statistics, census data, other public documents, analysis of and by agencies, community contacts, and observations.
3. records data in a standardized, systematic, and concise form.

In addition to the above, the nurse specialist—
1. plans, implements, and evaluates data collection, using advanced methodologies such as surveys, sampling techniques, and instrument construction.
2. uses principles of epidemiology, demography, and biometry, and relevant social, behavioral, and physical sciences to structure data collections.

The nurse generalist—

1. in partnership with the family and individual, collects health-related data in the following areas:
   a. health histories.
   b. physical assessment.
   c. growth and development.
   d. mental and emotional status.
   e. family dynamics.
   f. economic, environmental, legal, and political factors affecting health.
   g. cultural and religious factors affecting health.
   h. knowledge, satisfaction, and motivation regarding health.
   i. strengths that maintain and promote health.
   j. risk factors that affect health.
2. records data in a timely, standardized, systematic, and concise form.

In addition to the above, the nurse specialist—

1. designs, manages, and evaluates the data collection system.
2. serves as a consultant to the nurse generalist in implementation of the data collection system.

Outcome Criteria

1. The community, family, and individual participate in the data collection process.
2. The data are synthesized and recorded in a standardized and retrievable form.
3. The data are accurate and current.

Standard III. Diagnosis

THE NURSE ANALYZES DATA COLLECTED ABOUT THE COMMUNITY, FAMILY, AND INDIVIDUAL TO DETERMINE DIAGNOSES.

Rationale

Nursing's logical basis for intervention rests on identification of diagnoses that guide health promotion, illness reduction, and rehabilitation.

Structure Criteria

The practice setting provides opportunities for—

1. validation of diagnoses by colleagues, community, family, and individual.
2. exchange of information and research findings regarding the premises underlying diagnoses.
3. access to resources and relevant professional development programs.
4. systematic recording of diagnoses for the community, family, and individual.

Process Criteria

COMMUNITY

The nurse generalist collaborates with the nurse specialist in formulating diagnoses.

The nurse specialist—

1. in partnership with the community, interprets and analyzes data to formulate diagnoses regarding—
   a. inaccessible and unavailable services.
   b. mortality and morbidity rates.
   c. communicable disease rates.
   d. specific populations at risk for physical or emotional problems.
   e. health promotion needs for specific populations.
   f. community dysfunction.
   g. environmental hazards.
2. reviews and revises diagnoses based on subsequent data collection.

FAMILY AND INDIVIDUAL

The nurse generalist—

1. in partnership with the family and individual, interprets and analyzes collected data to formulate diagnoses.
2. reviews and revises diagnoses based on subsequent data collection.

In addition to the above, the nurse specialist—

1. serves as a consultant to the nurse generalist in formulating and revising diagnoses.
2. tests the appropriateness and relevancy of diagnoses to practice.

Outcome Criteria

1. The diagnoses are validated by the community, family, and individual when appropriate.
2. The diagnoses are accepted by colleagues as relevant and significant.
3. The diagnoses are recorded in a manner that facilitates planning, intervention, and evaluation, and provides direction for research.

Standard IV. Planning

AT EACH LEVEL OF PREVENTION, THE NURSE DEVELOPS PLANS THAT SPECIFY NURSING ACTIONS UNIQUE TO CLIENT NEEDS.

Rationale

Planning guides community health nursing interventions and facilitates achieving desired outcomes. Plans are based on the nursing diagnoses and contain specific goals and interventions.

Structure Criteria
1. The practice setting provides the necessary resources for the development of plans derived from the nursing diagnoses.
2. Within the practice setting, mechanisms exist for plans to be recorded, retrieved, updated, and communicated.
3. The practice setting has a written system for establishing priorities for services to communities, families, and individuals.

Process Criteria

COMMUNITY

The nurse generalist collaborates with the specialist in establishing priorities for services provided to the community.

The nurse specialist—
1. in partnership with the community, devises community-focused plans that are based on the nursing diagnosis and—
   a. reflect relevant theoretical concepts and research findings.
   b. include measurable goals and behavioral objectives with an expected date of accomplishment.
   c. identify a sequence of actions for achieving goals.
   d. propose contingency actions.
   e. list resources necessary to accomplish the plan.
   f. estimate the cost and benefits of the plan.
2. revises the plan as goals and objectives are achieved or changed.
3. records the plan in a standardized, systematic, and concise form.

FAMILY AND INDIVIDUAL

The nurse generalist—
1. in partnership with the family and individual, devises plans that are based on the nursing diagnosis and—
   a. reflect relevant theoretical concepts and research findings as a basis for the proposed plan.
   b. include measurable goals and behavioral objectives with an expected date of accomplishment.
   c. identify a sequence of actions for achieving goals and behavioral objectives.
   d. propose contingency actions.
   e. list resources necessary to accomplish the plan.
   f. estimate the cost and benefits of the plan.
2. revises the plan as goals and objectives are achieved or changed.
3. records the plan in a standardized, systematic, and concise form.

In addition to the above, the nurse specialist—
1. serves as a consultant to the nurse generalist in the planning process.
2. coordinates the establishment of priorities for provision of services to the family and individual.

Outcome Criteria
1. The community, family, and individual participate in the planning process.
2. The plan is reflective of the nursing diagnoses.
3. The plan exists in a concise, standardized, and retrievable form.
4. The plan shows evidence of revision as goals and objectives are achieved or changed.

Standard V. Intervention

THE NURSE, GUIDED BY THE PLAN, INTERVENES TO PROMOTE, MAINTAIN, OR RESTORE HEALTH, TO PREVENT ILLNESS, AND TO EFFECT REHABILITATION.

Rationale
The nurse implements the plan to achieve goals and objectives. Participation of the community, family, and individual in the interventions is necessary to effect the desired outcomes.

Structure Criteria
1. The community health nurse is an identifiable and accessible health care provider.
2. Independent nursing interventions are encouraged within the practice setting.
3. Staffing patterns in the community health care setting are determined by the documented health care needs of the population served.
4. A mechanism exists for reviewing and revising the staffing patterns periodically.
5. Intervention skills are maintained and increased through professional development.
6. Nursing consultation is available.

Process Criteria

COMMUNITY
The nurse generalist collaborates with the nurse specialist in appropriate interventions.

The nurse specialist—
1. in partnership with the community, implements appropriate programs to achieve health goals.
2. collaborates with a variety of others, including health care providers, community leaders, and organizations, to implement programs and develop resources necessary to meet identified needs.
3. ensures that the community is informed about its health, the resources of the health care delivery system, and other community systems that influence health.

4. reviews and revises interventions in accord with community response and statistical data.
5. formulates and influences health and social policies that affect the health of the community.

FAMILY AND INDIVIDUAL

The nurse generalist—
1. implements the interventions with the participation of the family and individual.
2. intervenes to treat physical and psychological responses to changes in health and developmental status.
3. collaborates with other health professionals to improve health and developmental status.
4. supervises ancillary personnel who provide care to families and individuals.
5. serves as a coordinator of services and an advocate for the family and individual to achieve health goals.
6. informs the family and individual regarding their health status and health care resources.
7. teaches the family and individual self-care concepts and skills, and assists in modifying the environment to encourage their use.
8. reviews and revises interventions based on individual and family response.

In addition to the above, the nurse specialist acts as a consultant to the nurse generalist in implementing the plan of action.

Outcome Criteria
1. The nursing interventions and client responses are recorded in a systematic, retrievable manner.
2. Nursing interventions are accepted by the community, family, and individual.
3. There is measurable evidence of progress toward goal achievement.

Standard VI. Evaluation

THE NURSE EVALUATES RESPONSES OF THE COMMUNITY, FAMILY, AND INDIVIDUAL TO INTERVENTIONS IN ORDER TO DETERMINE PROGRESS TOWARD GOAL ACHIEVEMENT AND TO REVISE THE DATA BASE, DIAGNOSES, AND PLAN.

Rationale
Nursing practice is a dynamic process that implies alterations in data, diagnoses, or plans previously made. The effectiveness of nursing care depends on the ongoing reassessment of community, family, and individual health, and on appropriate revision of the plan.

Structure Criteria

1. The nurse has access to information regarding changes in the overall client situation that would influence revision of the plan.
2. Supervision and consultation is available in the practice setting to assist the nurse in evaluating the effectiveness of nursing interventions and developing alternative plans when appropriate.
3. The practice setting provides a means for the community, family, or individual to participate in the evaluation process and revision of the nursing care plan.
4. The practice setting has in place a plan for program evaluations.

Process Criteria

COMMUNITY

The nurse generalist collaborates with the nurse specialist in evaluating community responses to interventions.

The nurse specialist—

1. plans for ongoing, timely, and comprehensive evaluation of the outcomes of interventions.
2. uses baseline and current data in measuring progress toward goal achievement.
3. validates observations, insights, and new data with colleagues and community members.
4. in partnership with the community, revises priorities, goals, and interventions to reflect the results of the evaluation process.
5. clearly documents evaluation results and revisions of the plan.
6. conducts program evaluation of the structure, process, and outcomes of health care that may include the following components:
   a. cost-benefit analysis.
   b. recording system.
   c. quality of interventions.
   d. immediate and long-term outcomes, both intended and unintended.
7. communicates the results of program evaluation to other program planners and decision makers.
8. conducts evaluation research with appropriate consultation.

FAMILY AND INDIVIDUAL

The nurse generalist—

1. plans for the ongoing, timely, and comprehensive evaluation of the outcomes of interventions.
2. uses baseline and current data in measuring progress toward goal achievement.
3. validates observations, insights, and new data with colleagues, families, and individuals.
4. in partnership with the family and individual, revises priorities, goals, and

interventions to reflect the results of the evaluation process.
5. clearly documents evaluation results and revisions of the plan.
6. participates in the evaluation of care through record audit and other methods of peer review.

In addition to the above, the nurse specialist—
1. serves as a consultant to nurse generalists in evaluating the impact of interventions with the family and individual.
2. evaluates the system for setting priorities for services to families and individuals.

Outcome Criteria
1. Data base, diagnosis, and plans are revised based on evaluation.
2. The community, family, and individual participate in the evaluation process and revision of the plan.
3. Program evaluation is used in making program decisions.
4. Evaluation of interventions is documented in a manner that contributes to the effectiveness of nursing actions and to research.

Standard VII. Quality Assurance and Professional Development

THE NURSE PARTICIPATES IN PEER REVIEW AND OTHER MEANS OF EVALUATION TO ASSURE QUALITY OF NURSING PRACTICE. THE NURSE ASSUMES RESPONSIBILITY FOR PROFESSIONAL DEVELOPMENT AND CONTRIBUTES TO THE PROFESSIONAL GROWTH OF OTHERS.

Rationale
Scientific, cultural, social, and political changes in society require a commitment from the nurse to the continuing pursuit of knowledge to enhance professional growth. Continuing education and evaluation of nursing practice by peer review and other methods of quality assurance are ways to ensure excellence.

Structure Criteria
1. A mechanism for peer review is provided within the practice setting.
2. Nurses are represented on quality assurance teams that evaluate health care outcomes.
3. Policies exist within the practice setting that provide opportunities for continuing education.
4. Opportunities are provided for participation in professional organization activities.
5. Opportunities for self-evaluation and evaluation by communities, families, and individuals are provided in the practice setting.

Process Criteria

The nurse—

1. initiates and participates in the peer review process.
2. participates in professional development programs, such as in-service sessions, conventions, and formal academic study, to increase knowledge and skills.
3. assists others in identifying areas of educational needs, and communicates new knowledge to others.
4. incorporates appropriate changes in his or her own practice suggested by self-evaluation, clients' evaluations, peer review, and professional development activities.
5. demonstrates professional responsibility by participation in appropriate professional organizations.

Outcome Criteria

The nurse—

1. meets continuing education requirements for relicensure and recertification as appropriate.
2. incorporates new information and methods into practice.
3. participates in self-evaluation, the peer review process, and professional development programs.
4. participates in professional and community organizations.

Standard VIII. Interdisciplinary Collaboration

THE NURSE COLLABORATES WITH OTHER HEALTH CARE PROVIDERS, PROFESSIONALS, AND COMMUNITY REPRESENTATIVES IN ASSESSING, PLANNING, IMPLEMENTING, AND EVALUATING PROGRAMS FOR COMMUNITY HEALTH.

Rationale

Community health nursing practice requires planning and sharing with others in the community to promote health for the community, family, and individual. Through the collaborative process, the special abilities of others are used to communicate, plan, solve problems, and evaluate services.

Structure Criteria

1. Opportunities for interdisciplinary collaboration are provided within the practice setting.
2. Opportunities for participation with other colleagues in policy making and planning for the agency and the community are encouraged within the practice setting.

Process Criteria

The nurse—

1. participates in the formulation of goals, plans, and decisions.

2. recognizes and respects the contributions of professional colleagues and community representatives.
3. consults with colleagues as needed.
4. articulates nursing and public health knowledge and skills to others.
5. collaborates with other disciplines in teaching, supervision, and research.

Outcome Criteria
1. The nurse is an integral member of the interdisciplinary team.
2. Nursing practice plans reflect interdisciplinary collaboration.

Standard IX. Research

THE NURSE CONTRIBUTES TO THEORY AND PRACTICE IN COMMUNITY HEALTH NURSING THROUGH RESEARCH.

Rationale
Improvement of community health nursing practice depends on the commitment of the nurse to the continuing development and refinement of knowledge through research.

Structure Criteria
1. Resource material regarding research in community health nursing and related disciplines is accessible in the practice setting.
2. The incorporation of research findings in the provision of care to communities, families, and individuals is encouraged within the practice setting.
3. Agency policy is supportive of research in community health nursing, as indicated by the following:
   a. The agency serves as a site for research related to community health nursing by its personnel and/or external researchers.
   b. The agency recognizes and supports research initiatives of community health nurses on its staff.
   c. A formal mechanism exists within the agency for review of proposed research studies, including their ethical implications.

Process Criteria
The nurse generalist—
1. critically reads and evaluates reported research for applicability of findings to practice.
2. identifies practice-related problems for investigation.
3. contacts appropriate persons who are prepared to initiate the research process and implement research projects.
4. participates in agency-based research projects under the supervision of qualified nurse researchers.

The nurse specialist, with appropriate consultation and/or collaboration with doctorally prepared researchers—

1. refines researchable problems relevant to community health nursing theory and practice.
2. participates in the design of research studies appropriate to the agency setting.
3. prepares proposals for support of research projects from internal and external sources.
4. participates in all phases of project implementation, including data collection, analysis, and interpretation.
5. ensures that research findings are accurately reported and disseminated.
6. serves as a resource to the nurse generalist in the identification and evaluation of research findings for application to community health nursing practice.

Outcome Criteria

1. Research activities occur within the practice setting.
2. The practice of community health nursing reflects the incorporation of currently validated findings from research.
3. The knowledge base of community health nursing is continually augmented and updated by the findings of relevant research studies.

GLOSSARY

BIOMETRICS. The statistical study of biological observations and phenomena.

CLIENT. A community, group, family, or individual for whom the nurse is providing formally specified services as sanctioned by nursing practice acts.

COMMUNITY. A social group determined by geographical boundaries and/or common values and interests. It functions within a particular social structure, exhibits and creates norms and values, and establishes social institutions. (This definition is adapted from a work of the World Health Organization.[15])

COMMUNITY HEALTH NURSE SPECIALIST. A licensed professional nurse who, through study and supervised practice at the graduate level (master's or doctoral), has become an expert in the knowledge and practice of community health nursing.

COMMUNITY HEALTH NURSING. A synthesis of nursing practice and public health practice applied to promoting and preserving the health of populations. Health promotion, health maintenance, health education and management, coordination, and continuity of care are used in a holistic approach to the management of the health care of individuals, families, and groups in a community. (This definition is adapted from *A Conceptual Model of Community Health Nursing.*[16])

DEMOGRAPHY. The science dealing with social statistics concerning such topics as health, disease, births, and mortality.

FAMILY. A formal social living unit or group of persons who typically are related to each other and live in one home.

GENERALIST. A licensed professional nurse who has a baccalaureate in nursing and has demonstrated expertise in community health nursing practice.

HEALTH. The state of complete physical, mental, and social well-being; not merely the absence of disease or infirmity.

INTERVENTION. An action taken by the nurse alone or in partnership with the community to promote health or to treat a health problem. Nursing actions are carried out independently in the autonomous domain of nursing practice. They may also be carried out in collaboration with other public health professionals.

LEVELS OF PREVENTION

PRIMARY. Measures that actively promote health, prevent illness, and provide specific protection.

SECONDARY. Early diagnosis and prompt interventions to limit disabilities.

TERTIARY. Measures that reduce impairments and disabilities, minimize suffering caused by departures from good health, and promote the client's adjustment to immediate conditions; rehabilitation activities.

NURSING DIAGNOSIS. A name, taxonomy label, or summarizing group of words that conveys a nursing assessment conclusion regarding actual or potential health problems of a client. A nursing diagnosis involves a clinical judgment that the health or illness problem being addressed is one that the nurse has legal authority to treat.

OUTCOME CRITERIA. Criteria that focus on the end results of nursing care; a measurable change in the state of health of the community, family, or individual; the end product of a professional process; a change in the environment or in the attitude of the client toward health care.

PARTNERSHIP. Two or more individuals or organizations associated in a joint venture.

PEER REVIEW. The process by which nurses actively engaged in the practice of nursing appraise the quality of nursing care in a given situation in accordance with established standards of practice.

POPULATION. The collection of individuals in a geographically defined area, or a group of individuals within the community (such as school students, workers in industry, or persons of similar age).

PRIMARY HEALTH CARE. Essential health care made universally accessible to individuals and families in the community by means acceptable to them, through their full participation, and at a cost that the community and country can afford. It forms an integral part both of the country's health system (of which it is the nucleus) and of the overall social and economic development of the community. (This definition is adapted from a work of the World Health Organization.[17])

PROCESS CRITERIA. Criteria that describe the major sequence of events and activities in the practice of community health nurses in the delivery of patient care.

PUBLIC HEALTH NURSING. A synthesis of the body of knowledge from the public health sciences and professional nursing theories for the purpose of improving the health of the entire community. This goal lies at the heart of primary prevention and health promotion, and is the foundation for public health nursing practice. (This definition is adapted from a work of the American Public Health Association's Public Health Nursing Section.[18])

QUALITY ASSURANCE. Activities to estimate and increase the level of excellence in the alteration of the health status of consumers, attained through review of providers' performance of diagnostic, therapeutic, prognostic, or other health care activities.

STANDARD. A norm that expresses an agreed-upon level of performance that has been developed to characterize, measure, and provide guidance for achieving excellence in practice.

STRUCTURE CRITERIA. Criteria that focus on the environment and its resources. They include consideration of the purpose of the institution, agency, or program, and its legal authority to carry out its mission; organizational characteristics; physical resources and management; qualifications of health professionals and other workers; physical facilities and equipment; and status with regard to accreditation, certification, or approval by appropriate voluntary or governmental bodies.

REFERENCES

1. American Nurses Association. *A Plan for Implementation of the Standards of Nursing Practice.* Kansas City, Mo.: the Association, 1975, 4.

2. American Nurses Association. *Standards of Nursing Practice.* Kansas City, Mo.: the Association, 1973.

3. American Nurses Association. *Standards of Community Health Nursing Practice.* Kansas City, Mo.: the Association, 1973.

4. American Nurses Association. *A Plan for Implementation of the Standards of Nursing Practice.*

5. American Nurses Association. *Nursing: A Social Policy Statement.* Kansas City, Mo.: the Association, 1980.

6. American Nurses Association. *Standards of Nursing Practice.*

7. American Nurses Association. *Code for Nurses with Interpretive Statements.* Kansas City, Mo.: the Association, 1985.

8. American Nurses Association. *A Conceptual Model of Community Health Nursing.* Kansas City, Mo.: the Association, 1980.

9. American Nurses Association. *A Guide for Community-Based Nursing Services.* Kansas City, Mo.: the Association, 1985.

10. American Nurses Association. *The Scope of Practice of the Primary Health Care Nurse Practitioner.* Kansas City, Mo.: the Association, 1985.

11. American Nurses Association. *Community-Based Nursing Services: Innovative Models.* Kansas City, Mo.: the Association, 1986.

12. Milbank Memorial Fund Commission. *Higher Education for Public Health: A Report.* Nantucket, Mass.: Prodist, 1976, 3.

13. World Health Organization. *Alma-Ata 1978—Primary Health Care: Report of the International Conference on Primary Health Care, Alma-Ata, U.S.S.R.* Geneva, Switzerland: the Organization, 1978.

14. *Ibid.*

15. *Ibid.*

16. American Nurses Association. *A Conceptual Model of Community Health Nursing,* 2.

17. World Health Organization, *op. cit.*

18. American Public Health Association. *The Definition and Role of Public Health Nursing in the Delivery of Health Care.* Washington, D.C.: the Association, 1980.

Public Health Nursing: Scope and Standards of Practice

APPENDIX C. SCOPE AND STANDARDS OF PUBLIC HEALTH NURSING (1999)

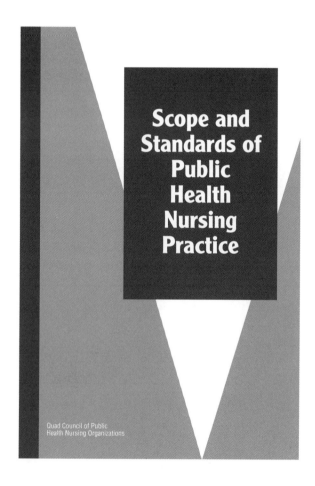

Scope and Standards of Public Health Nursing Practice

Quad Council of Public Health Nursing Organizations

SCOPE and STANDARDS
of
Public Health Nursing Practice

Quad Council of
Public Health Nursing Organizations

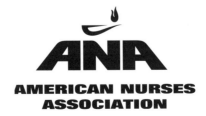

AMERICAN NURSES
ASSOCIATION

CONTENTS

INTRODUCTION

Since its beginnings in 1893 under the leadership of Lillian Wald, public health nursing has been a critical component of the country's health care system. Throughout the decades, this professional nursing specialty has been driven by the health needs of communities and populations.

At the turn of the twentieth century, public health nursing played a dominant role in the fight against diphtheria, smallpox, measles, and other communicable diseases. In the twenty-first century, public health nursing is positioned to embrace such challenges as bioterrorism, teen pregnancy, environmental hazards, chronic diseases, HIV/AIDS, and many others. Public health nursing has always responded to the priority health needs of society by serving individuals, families, groups, or entire communities and populations.

Current practice for many staff public health nurses aims primarily at health promotion and protection services for individuals. The practice of other public health nurses primarily focuses on populations. Because future public health services will be driven by local community needs, resources, and preferences of the people, all public health nurses must have a broad range of population-focused skills to be strong public health team partners.

The overall goal is to prepare the public health nursing workforce for this change, to be ready to make the necessary shift in practice. The challenge is to develop this capacity in a manner that builds on the strengths of the current public health nursing workforce, yet expands the knowledge base and skills required for public health nurses to be effective in dealing with contemporary and emerging issues within a rapidly changing society.

In view of these trends, the leaders of the Quad Council of Public Health Nursing Organizations, which represents nurses involved in population-focused and community-oriented nursing practice, collaborated to provide this *Scope and Standards of Public Health Nursing Practice*. The quad council comprises the American Nurses Association (ANA) Council for Community, Primary, and Long-Term Care Nursing Practice; the American Public Health Association Public Health Nursing Section; the Association of Community Health Nursing Educators; and the Association of State and Territorial Directors of Nursing.

SCOPE OF PUBLIC HEALTH NURSING PRACTICE

Public health nursing is the practice of promoting and protecting the health of populations using knowledge from nursing, social, and public health sciences (American Public Health Association, Public Health Nursing Section 1996). Public health nursing is population-focused, community-oriented nursing practice. The goal of public health nursing is the prevention of disease and disability for all people through the creation of conditions in which people can be healthy.

Public health nurses most often partner with nations, states, communities, organizations, and groups, as well as individuals, in completing health assessment, policy development, and assurance activities. Public health nurses practice in both public and private agencies. Some public health nurses may have responsibility for the health of a geographic or enrolled population, such as those covered by a health department or capitated health system, whereas others may promote the health of a specific population, for example, those with HIV/AIDS.

Public health nurses assess the needs and strengths of the population, design interventions to mobilize resources for action, and promote equal opportunity for health. Strong, effective organizational and political skills must complement their nursing and public health expertise.

Tenets of Public Health Nursing

The Quad Council of Public Health Nursing Organizations (1997) developed the following eight tenets of public health nursing to advance the public health nursing goal of promoting and protecting the health of the population.

1. **Population-based assessment, policy development, and assurance processes are systematic and comprehensive**. The client or unit of care is the population. Each process includes consideration of the community capacity, personal or lifestyle health practices, human biology, health services, and social, economic, physical, and environmental factors as they affect the population's health.

The assessment process includes a review of the needs, strengths, and expectations of all of the people and is guided by epidemiological methods. Policies are derived from assessment, are developed with a view toward the priorities set by the people, and consider subpopulations or communities whose health is at greatest risk, as well as the effectiveness of interventions and program options in influencing the health goals of the people. Interventions and programs are assured through direct provision of services by public health nurses, through regulation, or by encouraging the actions of other health care professionals or organizations, and focus on availability, acceptability, access, and quality of services.

2. **All processes must include partnering with representatives of the people.** This assures that the interpretation of the data, policy decisions, and planning of intervention strategies reflect the perspectives, priorities, and values of the people. By emphasizing representation from multiple communities, decisions are made with consideration of what is in the best interest of all.

3. **Primary prevention is given priority**. Primary prevention includes health promotion and health protection strategies. The practice of public health nursing places emphasis on primary prevention in all assessment, policy development, and assurance processes.

4. **Intervention strategies are selected to create healthy environmental, social, and economic conditions in which people can thrive.** Although all nurses are concerned about the environment in which individual clients live, public health nurses concentrate on interventions aimed at improving environments to benefit the health of the population. Interventions include educational, community development, social engineering, as well as policy development and enforcement strategies. Interventions tend to emerge from the political or community participation process and result in governmental policies and laws, administrative rules, and budget priorities. Interventions also emerge from policy and resource control mechanisms within public or private organizations. Some interventions will support functions and systems that promote

health, whereas others will protect the health of the people by prohibiting harmful practices.

5. **Public health nursing practice includes an obligation to actively reach out to all who might benefit from an intervention or service.** Often, those most likely to benefit are those who are the most marginal recipients. Because risk factors are not randomly distributed in the population, the health of some subpopulations may be more vulnerable to the development of disease and disability, or they may have more difficulty accessing and using interventions or services. Thus high-risk subpopulations or communities may need special outreach or programs so they can achieve an improvement in their risk status or health. Public health nursing focuses on the whole population and not solely on those who present themselves for services.

6. **The dominant concern and obligation is for the greater good of all of the people or the population as a whole.** Because the unit of care for this specialty is the population, consideration of what is in the best interest of the whole takes priority over the best interest of an individual or a group. Public health nurses also promote the health of individuals, but this responsibility is secondary to their obligation to promote the health of the population. Public health nurses recognize that it may not be possible to meet identified individual needs when those needs conflict with other priority health goals that benefit the whole population.

7. **Stewardship and allocation of available resources supports the maximum population health benefit gain.** This includes providing needed information to members of the population and leaders for the optimal use of available resources for the best overall improvement in the health of the entire population. Information should include scientific data on potential outcomes of various policy decisions, as well as the cost-benefit or cost-effectiveness of potential intervention strategies.

8. **The health of the people is most effectively promoted and protected through collaboration with members of other professions and organizations.** Creating conditions in which people can be healthy is an extremely complex, resource-

intense process. Public health nurses join with appropriate experts from multiple professions and organizations in efforts to improve population health.

Public health nursing practice includes providing leadership to assure that all of the people have their collective and individual nursing needs met. This includes (a) collaborating with other nurses in developing public policies that assure an adequate supply of well-prepared nurses to work in all health settings, (b) developing and enforcing public and organizational policies that assure access to quality nursing services, and (c) supporting nursing research and evaluation to promote quality of care by all nurses. Public health nurses also assure the availability of care to individuals and families in the community (community-based care) when their health condition creates a risk to the health of the population. In this situation, community-based care is a public health nursing strategy that directly benefits the whole population by reducing exposure to risk factors.

Examples of Public Health Nursing Activities

Examples of public health nursing activities include the following (American Public Health Association 1996):

1. Evaluating health trends and risk factors of population groups and helping to determine priorities for targeted interventions.

2. Working with communities or specific population groups within the community to develop public policy and targeted health promotion and disease prevention activities.

3. Participating in assessing and evaluating health care services to ensure that people are informed of available programs and services and assisted in the utilization of those services.

4. Providing essential input to interdisciplinary programs that monitor, anticipate, and respond to public health problems in population groups.

5. Providing health education, care management, and primary care to individuals and families who are members of vulnerable populations and high-risk groups.

Distinguishing Public Health Nursing from Other Nursing Specialties

Public health nursing is distinguished from other nursing specialties through its adherence to all eight tenets of public health nursing, with the overall goal of promoting and protecting the health of the entire population by creating conditions in which people can be healthy. Nurses who practice in other specialties may address some or all of these tenets. However, members of other nursing specialties may not always incorporate all eight tenets into their nursing practice.

It is not the location of care but the focus of care that distinguishes public health nursing from other specialty areas. Historically, most of public health and community nursing practice occurred outside the walls of acute care institutions. This led to a common definition of public health and community health nursing as nursing care based, or located, in the community, outside the acute care institution. Although the location of care may be the same, public health nursing is not equivalent to community-based nursing because the recipient of care differs.

Table 1 shows that public health nurses work with the intended beneficiary (or his or her representative) of their care. For public health nurses, the beneficiary usually is a population, but could also include an individual or family as the focus. The public health nurse completes a comprehensive assessment, uses scientific methods to guide data collection and interpretation, and shares the collected data with representatives of the population.

For public health nursing practice, data from assessment of individuals and families can only be aggregated to the whole population when biostatistical approaches have determined that the individuals or families are truly representatives of the whole. Because a population may contain many subpopulations or communities whose values, beliefs, traditions, and cultures differ, it is important that the public health nurse seek assistance in ascertaining the meaning of collected data from each of those subpopulations or communities.

For public health nursing, the assessment process leads to development of plans to intervene for identified health concerns (Table 2). Planning for public health nursing involves the development of policies with consideration of the expertise of the public health

Table 1. Assessment Activities of Public Health Nursing

Population Focus	Individual Focus
Conduct assessments in partnership with representatives of the population in collaboration with other health care or public health professionals.	Conduct assessments with individuals or families.
Scope of assessment guided by epidemiological methods and scientific knowledge with consideration of all of the determinants of health, population values, beliefs, and meaning of health.	Scope of assessment guided by nursing knowledge to include the individual's or family's living environment, lifestyle, coping, support relationships, neighborhood, economic status, health status, care access, and other factors that might have a significant impact on health outcomes.
Data are interpreted on the basis of scientific information with consideration of multiple communities' meaning of the data and shared with policymakers.	Data and scientific interpretation are shared with the individual family so that they can use that information in making decisions.

nurses and the preferences of the population. If the public health nurse is focusing on the individual and family, their preferences and needs are supported in program development.

Public health nursing activities focus on assuring that the population has access to needed quality programs and services (Table 3).

Ethical Responsibilities

Nurses in public health nursing practice accept the ethical standards explicit in the *Code for Nurses with Interpretive Statements* (ANA

Table 2. Policy Development Activities of Public Health Nursing

Population Focus	Individual Focus
Assist elected representatives or organizational managers in developing policies and plans to address health concerns.	Assist individuals or families in developing plans to meet their health concerns.
Recommend strategies to meet identified population needs.	Recommend interventions or therapeutics that can meet identified needs.
Recommend to policymakers the need for members of multiple communities to be addressed to assure that policymakers are aware of the multiple needs and perspectives of various communities.	Facilitate networking of individuals or families with similar needs and support their efforts in program development.
Advocate for issues or health problems, intervention strategies, and the whole population, ensuring the best potential to improve the health of the people addresses their preferences.	Act as an advocate for a specific individual or family.

1985). Nurses who work with populations may encounter situations in which human rights and freedom are in jeopardy. Therefore, it is important that the rights of populations be acknowledged. These rights include the right to be autonomous, the right to make informed decisions, and the right to pursue conditions that promote their health.

After clear dialogue, due consideration, and an opportunity to question, a competent population has the right to make decisions about its health policies and programs without coercion. Competent populations have the right to refrain from or pursue health care recommendations when their decisions do not affect the health and well-being of other populations. In the event that conflicts arise regarding the best practices of public health nursing and the wish of

Table 3. Assurance Activities of Public Health Nursing

Population Focus	Individual Focus
Assist populations in implementation and evaluation of their plans.	Assist individuals or families in implementation and evaluation of their plans.
Assure the implementation of the developed population-focused policies, including interventions and programs delivered by both public health nurses and other health care professionals or organizations.	Provide holistic care to individuals or families in collaboration with other health and social service providers.
Ensure program activities include those aimed at assuring the availability, acceptability, access to, and quality of needed services.	Participate in quality improvement activities of care provided by nurses and other personnel within their organization.

a population, the nurse should seek legal consultation, ethical consultation, or both, to determine the best course of action.

The purpose of public health nursing science is to enhance the health of populations. The duties or privileges of nurses have their origins in the rights of their clients. Nurses must recognize and establish their professional privileges in accordance with their populations' needs and rights. Nurses must be represented on ethics committees that make decisions that affect their populations' rights and the rights of nurses.

Education

The baccalaureate is the entry into practice for nursing where the goal of practice is the health of the public. Master's prepared public health nurses develop and evaluate programs and policy designed to prevent disease and promote health for populations at risk. Associate degree nurses and licensed practical nurses may appropriately practice in community settings where care is directed toward the health or illness of individuals, rather than populations.

GUIDELINES FOR USING THE STANDARDS

These standards were developed with consideration of the ANA's *Standards of Clinical Nursing Practice* (1998) and are to be used in conjunction with other documents, such as *Nursing's Social Policy Statement* (ANA 1995), the *Code for Nurses with Interpretive Statements* (ANA 1985), standards of nursing practice for a specific population, and the public health nursing statement of the American Public Health Association (1996).

These standards are designed to guide public health nursing practice and validate the quality of those professional services. These standards may be incorporated into systems of quality assurance to evaluate services and institute programs of peer review and performance appraisal. Within these standards are criteria that address professional performance, such as use of theory, professional development, interdisciplinary collaboration, and research. Accountability of the nurse to the population, the population's rights, and population advocacy are implicit throughout the standards. Finally, the nurse is responsible for considering all cultural aspects that could influence the population's health and program preferences.

STANDARDS OF CARE

Standard I. Assessment

The public health nurse assesses the health status of populations using data, community resources identification, input from the population, and professional judgment.

Measurement Criteria

1. The assessment is conducted in partnership with representatives of the population and in collaboration with other health care or public health professionals.

2. The scope and methods of the assessment are guided by epidemiological principles and scientific knowledge, and consider all of the determinants of health, population values, beliefs, meaning of health, and community resources and assets.

3. Relevant data used in the assessment are documented in a retrievable form.

4. The data collection process is systematic and organized.

Standard II. Diagnosis

The public health nurse analyzes collected assessment data and partners with the people to attach meaning to those data and determine opportunities and needs.

Measurement Criteria

1. Data are interpreted on the basis of scientific information with consideration of multiple communities' meaning of the data.

2. Data and interpretations are shared with policymakers and other partners.

3. Target populations are selected using a variety of information sources regarding risk and include trend data.

4. Opportunities and needs amenable to public health nursing interventions are identified.

5. Priorities are selected in partnership with the people from those opportunities and needs amenable to public health nursing.

6. Opportunities and needs are documented in a way that facilitates determination of expected outcomes.

Standard III. Outcomes Identification

The public health nurse participates with other community partners to identify expected outcomes in the populations and their health status.

Measurement Criteria

1. The levels of expected health status changes are identified for the individual, family, community, system, and population.

2. Outcomes are clearly stated, culturally appropriate, and documented in measurable terms.

3. Outcomes are supported by applicable guidelines, plans, and standards.

4. Outcomes are designed to reflect the contributions of the partners involved in the achievement of those outcomes.

5. Outcomes are attainable in relation to available resources.

6. Outcomes include a time estimate for attainment.

Standard IV. Planning

The public health nurse promotes and supports the development of programs, policies, and services that provide interventions that improve the health status of populations.

Measurement Criteria

1. Policy development reflects the goal of improving the health of the population.

2. Representatives of the population, such as community groups and consumers, are assisted in developing plans that address

health needs and concerns and consider the values, beliefs, and traditions of the whole population.

3. Recommended programs and intervention strategies meet the identified needs and consider new or enhanced services and opportunities to target at-risk populations.

4. Intervention strategies with the best potential for improving the health of the people are formulated.

5. Recommendations simultaneously consider the needs of the individual, family, and community, with priority given to plans that promote the greatest improvement in the health of the population.

6. The needs and preferences of the multiple communities that constitute the population are considered.

7. Key policymakers are informed of the impact of health regulations, budget decisions, and other factors on the health of the community.

8. All plans reflect the tenets of current public health nursing practice.

9. All plans, programs, and intervention strategies are documented.

Standard V. Assurance: Action Component of the Nursing Process for Public Health Nursing

The public health nurse assures access and availability of programs, policies, resources, and services to the population.

Measurement Criteria

1. Collaboration with other health and human services organizations promotes the availability of personnel and public health services for all the people, consistent with the needs and preferences of multiple communities.

2. The public health nurse monitors activities that focus on improving the availability and quality of health care providers and services.

3. Populations are assisted in the implementation of programs, policies, and services.

4. Clinical programs are implemented for specific at-risk populations.

5. All interventions are consistent with established policies, plans, and services.

6. Documentation includes records of all policies, plans, programs, and services.

7. Resources are directed toward groups identified as being at highest risk of disease and disability.

Standard VI. Evaluation

The public health nurse evaluates the health status of the population.

Measurement Criteria

1. Continuous and systematic data collection using epidemiological and scientific methods is used to determine the effectiveness of public health nursing interventions.

2. The population is assisted in developing the plans for evaluation.

3. Evaluation is systematic and ongoing, and may include monitoring activities.

4. The collected information is used to improve existing policies, programs, and services, and also is considered as a part of the next needs assessment.

5. The evaluation examines the effectiveness of all interventions, including the need for modification of interventions, in relation to outcomes.

6. Documentation reflects the evaluation processes and the population's responses to policies, plans, and interventions.

STANDARDS OF PROFESSIONAL PERFORMANCE

Standard I. Quality of Care

The public health nurse systematically evaluates the availability, accessibility, acceptability, quality, and effectiveness of nursing practice for the population.

Measurement Criteria

Quality of care for public health nursing involves examination of agencies and programs of public health nursing, as well as all of the nursing activities for the population.

1. The public health nurse participates in the scope of quality of care activities as appropriate to the nurse's position, education, and practice environment. Such activities may include the following:

   - Identification of aspects of policies, programs, and services important for quality monitoring.

   - Identification of indicators used to monitor quality and effectiveness of policies, programs, and services.

   - Collection of data to monitor the availability, accessibility, acceptability, quality, and effectiveness of policies, programs, and services.

   - Analysis of quality data to identify opportunities for improving policies, programs, and services.

   - Formulation of recommendations to improve policies, programs, and services or population health outcomes.

   - Implementation of activities to enhance the quality of policies, programs, and services.

   - Participation on interdisciplinary teams that evaluate policies, programs, and services.

   - Development of policies, programs, and services to improve quality of care.

2. The nurse uses the results of quality of care activities to initiate changes in practice.

3. The nurse uses the results of quality of care activities to initiate changes throughout the health care delivery system, as appropriate.

Standard II. Performance Appraisal

The public health nurse evaluates his or her own nursing practice in relation to professional practice standards and relevant statutes and regulations.

Measurement Criteria

1. The nurse engages in performance appraisal on a regular basis, identifying areas of strength as well as areas for professional and practice development and improvement.

2. The nurse seeks constructive feedback regarding his or her own practice.

3. The nurse takes action to achieve goals identified during the performance appraisal.

4. The nurse participates in peer review as appropriate.

5. The nurse's practice reflects knowledge of current professional practice standards, laws, and regulations.

Standard III. Education

The public health nurse acquires and maintains current knowledge and competency in public health nursing practice.

Measurement Criteria

1. The nurse participates in educational activities to maintain and enhance the knowledge and skills necessary to promote the health of the population for which the nurse has responsibility.

2. The public health nurse seeks professional development experiences that are consistent with the changing needs of the population for which the nurse has responsibility.

Standard IV. Collegiality

The public health nurse establishes collegial partnerships while interacting with health care practitioners and others, and contributes to the professional development of peers, colleagues, and others.

Measurement Criteria

1. The nurse shares knowledge and skills with colleagues.

2. The nurse provides peers and other colleagues with constructive feedback regarding their efforts to improve the health of the public.

3. The nurse interacts with colleagues to enhance the nurse's own public health nursing practice.

4. The nurse contributes to an environment that is conducive to the public health nursing student, other health care students, and other employees, as appropriate.

5. The nurse's activities contribute to a supportive and healthy work environment.

Standard V. Ethics

The public health nurse applies ethical standards in advocating for health and social policy, and delivery of public health programs to promote and preserve the health of the population.

Measurement Criteria

1. The nurse's practice is guided by the *Code for Nurses with Interpretive Statements* (ANA 1985).

2. The nurse identifies situations in which ethical dilemmas and concerns are present or human rights and freedoms are in jeopardy.

3. The nurse identifies gaps in health services and policy and collaborates to correct them.

4. The nurse seeks consultation, as needed, to determine the best course of action in response to ethical dilemmas and risks to human rights and freedoms, including those of the populations.

5. The nurse implements policies and programs in a nonjudgmental and nondiscriminatory manner sensitive to the needs of the population.

6. The nurse implements policies and programs in a manner that promotes, protects, and preserves autonomy, confidentiality, dignity, and human rights.

7. The nurse advocates for and assists the population in developing skills to advocate for itself.

Standard VI. Collaboration

The public health nurse collaborates with the representatives of the population and other health and human service professionals and organizations in providing for and promoting the health of the population.

Measurement Criteria

1. The nurse communicates with representatives of the population and other health and human services professionals regarding nursing's role in the promotion of health.

2. The nurse, with other health and human services professionals, consults with representatives of the population so that the population's values, beliefs, and needs are considered.

3. The nurse collaborates with representatives of the population and other health and human services professionals in formulating policies and plans.

Standard VII. Research

The public health nurse uses research findings in practice.

Measurement Criteria

1. The nurse utilizes the best available evidence, preferably research data, to develop policies, plans, and interventions.

2. The nurse uses programs, policies, and services substantiated by research as appropriate to the nurse's position, education, and practice environment.

3. The nurse participates in research activities as appropriate. Such activities may include the following:

   - Identification of opportunities and needs suitable for public health nursing research.

   - Participation in data collection.

   - Participation in an agency, organization, or community research committee or program.

   - Sharing of research activities with others.

   - Conducting research.

   - Critiquing research for application to practice.

   - Using research findings in the development of policies, plans, procedures, programs, and guidelines for population care.

Standard VIII. Resource Utilization

The public health nurse considers safety, effectiveness, and cost in the planning and delivery of public health services when using available resources, to ensure the maximum possible health benefit to the population.

Measurement Criteria

1. The nurse analyzes the effectiveness, efficiency, and cost of interventions, policies, and programs, and utilizes that information in allocating resources.

2. The nurse designs policies, programs, and services that focus on members of the population who can best benefit from the interventions, assuring no duplication of existing policies, programs, and services.

3. To promote the health of the population, the nurse advocates for policies that create new programs and services when gaps in service delivery or unequal distribution of resources are identified, and for policies that eliminate programs and services when they are no longer a priority.

4. The nurse interacts with representatives of the population and other health and social or human services professionals to plan, organize, and evaluate resource availability and utilization.

REFERENCES

American Nurses Association. 1985. *Code for Nurses with Interpretive Statements.* Washington, D.C.: American Nurses Association.

American Nurses Association. 1995. *Nursing's Social Policy Statement.* Washington, D.C.: American Nurses Association.

American Nurses Association. 1998. *Standards of Clinical Nursing Practice.* 2d ed. Washington, D.C.: American Nurses Association.

American Public Health Association, Public Health Nursing Section. 1996. Definition and role of public health nursing. Washington, D.C.: American Public Health Association.

Quad Council of Public Health Nursing Organizations. 1997. The Tenets of Public Health Nursing. Unpublished white paper.

GLOSSARY

Assessment—The regular and systematic collection, analysis, and dissemination of information on the health of the community, including statistics on health status, community health needs, and epidemiological and other studies of health problems.

Assurance—Assuring services necessary to achieve agreed upon goals are provided by encouraging actions by other entities (private or public), by requiring such action through regulation, or by providing services directly.

Community—A group of people who have common characteristics. Communities can be defined by location, race, ethnicity, age, occupation, interest in particular problems or outcomes, or other common bonds.

Community-based—Designates the location or site at which services or activities occur, but does not define the content of the service.

Community-oriented—Term commonly used to define the community as the focus of care.

Determinants of health—Social, economic, and health care factors that affect health and well-being independently, and in conjunction with each other, at the population or community level. Comprehensive factors involve relevant social, economic, environmental, behavioral, political, health, and health care indicators that describe the essential features of a social structure and system and the processes through which change occurs.

Epidemiology—The study of the distribution of determinants and antecedents of health and disease in human populations. The ultimate goal is to identify the underlying causes of a disease and then to apply findings to disease prevention and health promotion.

Opportunities and needs—Situations, conditions, disabilities, and issues that provide an occasion to positively affect the future health of a population or that are considered undesirable and likely to exist in the future.

Outcomes—Long-term objectives that define optimal, measurable future levels of health status, maximum acceptable levels of disease, injury or dysfunction, or prevalence of risk factors.

Partners—Associates in a common activity or interest that may include other members of interdisciplinary professional groups, community members, policymakers, and community institutions and organizations.

Policy development—Applying comprehensive public health scientific knowledge for decision making. Policy development includes a systematic course of action to establish priorities, determine effective strategies and interventions, and use community resources, including regulation and law, to achieve the community's goals.

Population-based public health services—Interventions aimed at disease prevention and health promotion that affect an entire population and extend beyond medical treatment by targeting underlying risk, such as tobacco, drug, and alcohol use; diet and sedentary lifestyles; and environmental factors.

Prevention—Anticipatory action taken to prevent the occurrence of an event or to minimize its effects after it has occurred.

Risk—A behavior or condition that, on the basis of scientific evidence or theory, is thought to influence susceptibility to a specific health problem.

Standards of care—Authoritative statements that describe a competent level of clinical nursing practice demonstrated through assessment, diagnosis, outcome identification, planning, implementation, and evaluation.

Standards of nursing practice—Authoritative statements that describe a level of care or performance common to the profession of nursing by which the quality of nursing practice can be judged.

Standards of clinical practice include both standards of care and standards of professional performance.

Standards of professional performance—Authoritative statements that describe a competent level of behavior in the professional role, including activities related to quality of care, performance appraisal, education, collegiality, ethics, collaboration, research, and resource utilization.

Tenet—An opinion, doctrine, or principle considered as being true by an individual, or especially by an organization.

INDEX

Pages in the 1986 *Standards of Community Health Nursing Practice* or the 1999 *Scope and Standards of Public Health Nursing Practice* are marked by the year in brackets: [1986] or [1999].

105

American Nurses Association (*continued*)
   Code of Ethics for Nurses with Interpretive
      Statements, 9, 34
      [1986] 58
      [1999] 86, 90, 97
   Nursing: Scope and Standards of Practice,
      vii, 13
   Nursing's Social Policy Statement, [1999]
      90
   Scope and Standards for Nurse
      Administrators, 10
   Standards of Nursing Practice, *vii*
      [1986] 56
      [1999] 90
American Nurses Credentialing Center,
   11
American Public Health Association
   (APHA), *viii*, 3
   [1999] 80, 90
Analysis. *See* Critical thinking, analysis,
   and synthesis
Anderson & Mcfarlane ecological model,
   50
Assessment, 6
   [1986] 59
   [1999] 81, 82, 84, 85, 86
   defined, 41
   collaboration and, 32
   data collection and, [1986] 61, 62
   evaluation and, 26
   planning and, 19
   population diagnosis and, 17
   standard of practice, 15–16
      [1999] 91
   step in nursing process, *vii*, 13
Association of Community Health
   Nursing Educators (ACHNE), 3, 4
   [1999] 80
Association of State and Territorial
   Directors of Nursing (ASTDN), 3
   [1999] 80
Assurance, 6
   [1999] 81, 88
   defined, 41
   standard of practice, [1999] 93–94
ASTDN ecological model, 50

B
Biometrics, 15
   [1986] 59
Body of knowledge, 5
   [1999] 80, 86
   assessment and, [1999] 91
   education and, 10, 29
      [1999] 96
   implementation and, 21
   outcomes identification and, 18
   planning and, 19
   population diagnosis and, 17
   professional practice evaluation and, 30
   quality of practice and, 27
   research and, 36
      [1986] 70, 71

C
Care recipient. *See* Patient
Care standards. *See* Standards of practice
Case management. *See* Coordination
Certification and credentialing, 11
   [1986] 59
   [1999] 89
   professional practice evaluation and, 30
   quality assurance and professional
      development, [1986] 69
   quality of practice and, 28
Client, 8
   See also Community health; Family
      health; Individual health;
      Population focus
Clinical settings. *See* Practice settings
Coalition building (defined), 41
Code of Ethics for Nurses with Interpretive
      Statements, 9, 34
   [1986] 58
   [1999] 86, 90, 97
   See also Ethics
Collaboration, 2, 5, 9, 11
   [1999] 83, 84, 86
   assessment and, [1999] 91
   assurance and, [1999] 93
   data collection and, [1986] 61
   defined, 41
   implementation and, 21
   interventions and, [1986] 65, 66

Economic issues. *See* Cost control

Education of populations, 5, 8
  [1999] 84
  planning and, 19
  regulatory activities and, 25
  resource utilization and, 37
  See also Health education and health
    promotion

Education of public health nurses, *viii, ix,*
    1, 2, 10–11
  [1986] 58–59
  [1999] 82, 88–89
  collaboration and, 32, 33
  collegiality and, 31
    [1999] 97
  interdisciplinary collaboration and,
    [1986] 70
  leadership and, 38
  quality assurance and professional
    development, [1986] 68, 69
  quality of practice and, 27
    [1999] 95
  research and, [1999] 99
  standard of professional performance,
    29
    [1999] 96–97
  See also Mentoring; Professional
    development

Emergency preparedness. *See*
    Preparedness

Environmental health, 2, 5, 6
  [1999] 81
  assessment and, 15
  coordination and, 22
  data collection and, [1986] 61, 62
  defined, 42
  diagnosis and, [1986] 63
  ethics and, 34
  health education and health promotion,
    23
  interventions and, [1986] 66
  outcomes identification and, 18
  quality of practice and, 28
  See also Practice environment

*Environmental Health Principles and
    Recommendations for Public Health
    Nursing,* 9

EPI ecological model, 50

Epidemiology, 5, 6, 10, 26
  [1986] 57, 59
  [1999] 82, 86
  assessment and, 15
    [1999] 91
  data collection and, [1986] 61
  defined, 42
  evaluation and, 26
    [1999] 94

Ethics, 2, 9–10
  [1986] 58
  [1999] 86–88
  advocacy and, 40
  assessment and, 15
  data collection and, [1986] 61
  outcomes identification and, 18
  quality of practice and, 27
  research and, [1986] 70
  standard of professional performance,
    34–35
    [1999] 97–98
  See also Code of Ethics for Nurses with
    Interpretive Statements; Laws,
    statutes, and regulations

Evaluation, 4
  [1986] 59
  [1999] 84, 88
  collaboration and, 32
  data collection and, [1986] 61
  diagnosis and, [1986] 63
  health education and health promotion,
  leadership and, 38
  planning and, 19
  quality of practice and, 27
  standard of practice, 26
    [1986] 66–68
    [1999] 94
  step in nursing process, *vii,* 13

Evidence (defined), 42

Evidence-based practice, 4, 6, 7, 9
  [1999] 85
  defined, 42
  education and, 29
  health education and health promotion,
    23
  implementation and, 21

leadership and, 39
outcomes identification and, 18
planning and, 19
quality of practice and, 27, 28
See also Research

F
Faith-based organizations, 1, 6, 7
Family health, 7
Financial issues. *See* Cost control

G
Generalist practice public health nursing,
    [1986] 58–59
    [1999] 88
    advocacy, 40
    assessment, 15
        [1999] 91
    assurance, [1999] 93–94
    collaboration, 32
        [1999] 98–99
    collegiality and professional
        relationships, 31
        [1999] 97
    consultation, 24
    coordination, 22
    data collection, [1986] 61–62
    diagnosis
        [1986] 62–63
        [1999] 91–92
    education, 10, 29
        [1986] 58, 59
        [1999] 96–97
    ethics, 34
        [1999] 97–98
    evaluation, 26
        [1986] 66–68
        [1999] 94
    health education and health promotion,
        23
    implementation, 21
    interdisciplinary collaboration, [1986]
        69–70
    intervention, [1986] 65–66
    leadership, 38
    outcomes identification, 18
        [1999] 92

planning, 19
    [1986] 63–65
    [1999] 92–93
population diagnosis and priorities, 17
professional practice evaluation, 30
    [1999] 96
quality assurance and professional
    development, [1986] 68–69
quality of practice, 27–28
    [1999] 95–96
regulatory activities, 25
research, 36
    [1986] 70–71
    [1999] 99
resource utilization, 37
    [1999] 100
theory, [1986] 60
See also Public health nursing;
    Advanced practice public health
    nursing
Genomics, 2, 9
Global health, 2, 3
Governmental agencies, 1, 3, 5, 7
    consultation and, 24
    population diagnosis and, 17
Guidelines, 14
    advocacy and, 40
    leadership and, 39
    outcomes identification and, [1999] 92
    professional practice evaluation and, 30
    quality of practice and, 27
    See also Standards of practice;
        Standards of professional
        performance

H
Health determinants. *See* Determinants
    of health
Health education and health
    promotion, 2, 4, 8
    [1986] 57
    interventions and, [1986] 66
    planning and, 19
    population diagnosis and, 17
    standard of practice, 23
Health maintenance organizations
    (HMOs), 7

research and, [1999] 99
resource utilization and, [1999] 100
standard of practice, [1986] 65–66

K
Knowledge base. *See* Body of knowledge

L
Laffrey & Kulbok ecological model, 51
Laws, statutes, and regulations, 9
  advocacy and, 40
  assessment and, 15
  collaboration and, 33
  data collection and, [1986] 62
  education and, 29
  ethics and, 34
  evaluation and,
  planning and, 19, 20
  planning and, [1999] 93
  professional practice evaluation and, 30
    [1999] 96
  See also Ethics; Regulatory activities
Leadership, 4
  [1999] 84
  coordination and, 22
  health education and health
    promotion, 23
  standard of professional performance,
    38–39
Licensing. *See* Certification and
    credentialing

M
Measurement criteria. *See* Criteria
Mentoring
  collegiality and, 31
  leadership and, 38
MN ecological model, 51
Morbidity and mortality, 9
  diagnosis and, [1986] 63
Multidisciplinary healthcare. *See* Inter-
    disciplinary health care
Multi-sector team
  collegiality and, 31
  defined, 42
  ethics and, 35

leadership and, 38, 39
planning and, 20
resource utilization and, 37
See also Collaboration; Health
    professionals; Interdisciplinary
    health care

N
*National Public Health Performance
    Standards*, 3, 4
Nursing care standards. *See* Standards
    of care
Nursing process
  quality of practice and, 27
  steps, *vii*, 13
  [1986] 56
  See also Standards of Practice
Nursing standards. *See* Standards of
    practice; Standards of professional
    performance

O
Outcomes, 7, 9
  [1999] 83
  advocacy and, 40
  coordination and, 22
  defined, 42
  diagnosis and, [1999] 92
  ethics and, 35
  evaluation and, 26
    [1986] 67
    [1999] 94
  interventions and, [1986] 65
  leadership and, 38
  planning and, 19
    [1986] 63
  population diagnosis and, 17
  quality assurance and professional
    development, [1986] 68
  resource utilization and, 37
  See also Outcomes identification
Outcomes identification
  standard of practice, 18
    [1999] 92
  step in nursing process, *vii*, 13
  See also Outcomes

Quality assurance and professional
 development
 standard of professional performance,
 [1986] 68–69
Quality of practice, 3
 [1986] 59
 [1999] 84, 88, 90
 evaluation and, [1986] 67
 resource utilization and, 37
 standard of professional performance,
 27–28
 [1999] 95–96

R

Recipient of care. *See* Patient
Referrals. *See* Collaboration; Coordination
Regulatory activities
 standard of practice, 25
 See also Laws, statutes, and regulations
Research, *viii, ix*, 1, 2, 6, 7
 [1986] 59
 [1999] 83, 84
 collaboration and, 32, 33
 diagnosis and, [1986] 63
 education and, 10, 29
 evaluation and, [1986] 67
 health education and health promotion,
 23
 interdisciplinary collaboration and,
 [1986] 70
 planning and, 19
 [1986] 64
 quality of practice and, 28
 standard of professional performance,
 36
 [1986] 70–71
 [1999] 99
 See also Evidence-based practice
Resource utilization, 8
 [1999] 81, 83
 assurance and, [1999] 94
 health education and health
 promotion, 23
 implementation and, 21
 interventions and, [1986] 65
 outcomes identification and, 18
 [1999] 92
 planning and, [1986] 64

standard of professional performance,
 37
 [1999] 100
Risk assessment,
 [1999] 84
 data collection and, [1986] 62
 diagnosis and, [1999] 91
 ethics and, 35
 outcomes identification and, 18
 planning and, 19
 population diagnosis and, 17
 resource utilization and, 37
Roles in public health nursing practice, 4

S

Safety assurance
 advocacy and, 40
 collegiality and, 31
 health education and health promotion,
 23
 implementation and, 21
 quality of practice and, 28
 resource utilization and, 37
 [1999] 100
Salmon ecological model, 51
Scientific findings. *See* Evidence-based
 practice; Research
*Scope and Standards of Public Health
 Nursing Practice* (1999), *vii*, 3, 77–104
*Scope and Standards for Nurse
 Administrators*, 10
Scope of practice, 1–11
 [1986] 56–59
 [1999] 81–89
Self care and self-management
 interventions and, [1986] 66
Settings. *See* Practice environment
Social justice (defined), 43
Specialty certification. *See* Certification
 and credentialing
Stakeholder (defined), 43
Standard (defined), 43
Standards of care
 origins, *vii*
 [1986] 56
 See also Standards of practice
Standards of Community Health Nursing
 (1986), *vii*, 53–75